"Amy Hammer separates menstrual facts from fiction in a way that is both friendly and approachable. Packed with crucial information you may have missed in health class, *Cycles* gives you everything you need to reclaim and embrace all the seasons of your cycle."

—**Amanda Laird, registered holistic nutritionist, author of *Heavy Flow: Breaking the Curse of Menstruation*, and host of the Heavy Flow Podcast**

"For menstruators, learning about our biology and the intricacies of our menstrual cycle is a crucial part of unlearning the stigma we've lived through and the misinformation we've maybe been exposed to. Periods are powerful, and with a deeper understanding of our bodily changes, we can make informed decisions to maximize our energies and capabilities according to our menstrual cycles. I love that this book is one step to help do that!"

—**Nadya Okamoto, author of *Period Power: A Manifesto for the Menstrual Movement***

"In *Cycles*, Amy J. Hammer has written a remarkably thorough, comprehensive, and accessible guide to the reproductive and sexual health of humans who menstruate. She situates menstrual cycles in context of cycles of life and seasons of nature in a way that enhances our understanding of menstruation. The text presents a finely tuned balance of the complexity and variety of individual cycles with commonalities across cycles and menstruators, with many helpful illustrations. Hammer explains medical terms for anatomy and for physiological processes clearly and concisely, without getting weighed down by jargon. *Cycles* can be read straight through or in sections of interest, then kept on the shelf as a reference for life."

—**Elizabeth A. Kissling, PhD, professor emerita of Gender, Women's, and Sexuality Studies, Eastern Washington University**

"Amy Hammer's *Cycles* is a modern update to understanding our menstrual cycles. The blend of history with modern-day science and thoughtful illustrations makes *Cycles* as interesting as a good novel."

—**Halley Strongwater, clinical herbalist and founder of Loam Earth**

"*Cycles* is the book you always wish you had about your cycle that breaks down the science and history behind menstruation and beyond in an accessible, easy-to-digest way, while offering no-nonsense tips to improve not only your menstrual health but overall health as well. After reading the book, it struck me just how little I knew about something I experience every month."

—**Auri Jackson, producer at Buzzfeed and writer, director, and producer of *The Spot***

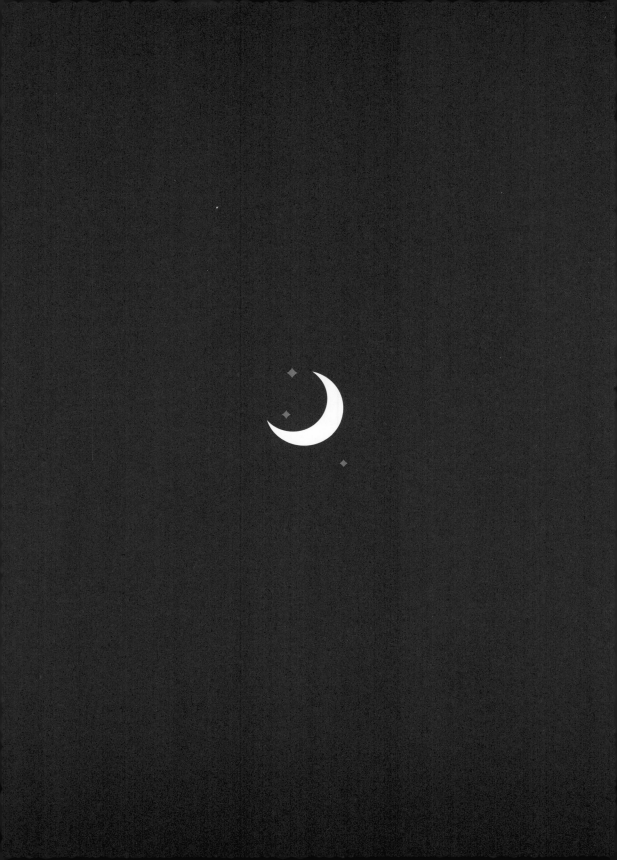

cycles

The Science of Periods, Why They Matter, and How to Nourish Each Phase

Amy J. Hammer, FNP

Illustrated by Fátima Bravo

Roost Books
An imprint of Shambhala Publications, Inc.
2129 13th Street
Boulder, Colorado 80302
www.roostbooks.com

The information presented in this book is for educational purposes only and
is not intended to diagnose or treat any health conditions. Please consult your
health practitioner regarding any specific health concerns and personal care.

Illustrations © 2023 by Fátima Bravo

Cover art: Fátima Bravo
Cover and interior design: Amy Sly

9 8 7 6 5 4 3 2 1

First Edition
Printed in Singapore

Shambhala Publications makes every effort to print on acid-free,
recycled paper.

Roost Books is distributed worldwide by Penguin Random House, Inc.,
and its subsidiaries.

Library of Congress Cataloging-in-Publication Data
Names: Hammer, Amy, author.
Title: Cycles: the science of periods, why they matter, and how to nourish each
phase / Amy J. Hammer; illustrated by Fatima Bravo.
Description: First edition. | Boulder, Colorado: Roost Books, [2023] |
Includes index.
Identifiers: LCCN 2021055757 | ISBN 9781611809060 (trade paperback)
Subjects: LCSH: Menstruation—Miscellanea. | Hormones. | Women—Health
and hygiene.
Classification: LCC RG163 .H36 2023 | DDC 618.172—dc23/eng/20211216
LC record available at https://lccn.loc.gov/2021055757

Dedicated to my mom, whose menstrual cycle education consisted of a book about periods slipped into her underwear drawer. Thank you for empowering me with information and talking openly with me about all of the transitions of life.

Contents

PART THREE

Exploring the Four Seasons of Life 187

Introduction

Many years ago, I was trying to learn how to surf while visiting a friend in Maui. After a few days learning in the whitewash and two-foot baby waves, we went to another spot with three- to four-foot waves. After paddling out and spending most of my time trying and failing (and flailing), I finally caught a ride. I made it pretty close to the shoreline, and then got back on my board, flipped it around, and as I started paddling back out, a set of much bigger waves rolled in. One after the other, waves crashed on me as I mistimed a duck dive under them on my board. I got stuck in a cycle of trying to paddle, getting crashed, and sputtering like I was in a washing machine. I was getting wrecked. Gasping and squinting through my burning saltwater-filled eyes, I was in a full-on fight with the ocean and, of course, I was losing miserably.

At the peak of my frustration, feeling a little panicked, I got off my board and found, to my embarrassment and relief, that I was standing in about five feet of water. I expected the ocean bottom to be full of coral or sharp rocks ready to cut my feet, but instead, it was sandy, and I felt its smooth rippled surface beneath my toes. I caught my breath and felt suddenly stable, rooted in the ground even while the waves still swelled and crashed around me. The reorientation was shocking and simple, and I felt like a completely happy fool.

It turns out I'm still not a good surfer. But I am a person who needs to consistently find solid, stable ground, especially when the waves around me feel especially choppy. When everything feels overwhelming and impossible, I need strategies that bring me back to myself and help me find peace. One of the ways I find consistent stability is through a daily walking habit. About a quarter-mile north of my home in the high desert, there is a large public park that runs up against national forestland. For the past ten years, I've walked through this park and the high desert mountains through all of the seasons and cyclic waves of both the desert and my life.

Through consistent attention and observation, my understanding of the seasons of the desert and my sense of home here have grown. The winter, a season of reflection and quiet, is a time of rest and then rebirth as it gives way to a surprisingly beautiful springtime marked by a feeling of renewal and unfolding. Spring swings into summer, a season that is unapologetically open and carefree. The fall is contemplative; a time when I notice each small shift in the air as the weather changes and as the flowers and leaves that regenerated so fully during the spring and summer part with their still-alive branches and cover the paths in dense layers of red, orange, and yellow, slowly but surely bringing back winter.

In the same way that I feel grounded and at home here in the desert because I pay close attention to its seasons and cycles, I invite you to root yourself in the seasons and cycles in the landscape that is your body. This book is meant to act as a "sandy bottom" for you to sink your feet into as you navigate your reproductive and overall health, your menstrual cycle, and each season of your life, which can at times feel as turbulent as the ocean waves.

In Part One, "Reclaiming Your Cycle," we'll talk about why the menstrual cycle matters in the context of evolutionary biology (hint, it has to do with the fact that the uterus is "choosy") and why it is considered a vital sign of health. We'll explore the fascinating history of hormones and the sex hormones that shape the menstrual cycle. In chapter three, you'll read about a physician who believed intellectual thought and higher education made menstruating people both "irritable and infertile" and you'll learn about the scientist who challenged him and proved him wrong. We'll discuss how the menstrual cycle affects how we process our experiences and how our lifestyle affects and shapes menstrual health. The end of Part One is about the history of contraception (goat bladder condoms, anyone?), reproductive science, and modern options for birth control including hormonal contraceptives, barriers methods like condoms, and fertility awareness-based methods.

Part Two, "The Four Seasons of Your Cycle," is a practical guide to supporting and understanding the menstrual cycle. Each phase of the cycle is explored as its own season with cycle-specific information. For example, we'll look at how prostaglandins and uterine blood flow influence period-related pain during the menstrual phase and how cultural ideals of femininity and self-policing contribute to PMS symptoms during the late luteal phase. Deeply nourishing recipes featuring foods that support overall well-being accompany each season along with self-care practices and diverse, full-body movements. The goal of this section is to provide accessible tools and information that you can return to again and again as you cycle through each phase every month.

In Part Three, "Exploring the Four Seasons of Life," we'll look at specific health challenges we face during menarche (the first menstrual cycle), the menstruating years, the menopausal transition, and the postmenopausal years. These chapters examine how our reproductive health shifts over time; for example, as adolescents, we're in a process of discovery and forming a relationship with our bodies, while the menstruating years are marked by having children or not and by our work. The menopausal transition is a significant time of change, fluctuation, and recalibration. Through examining the physiology and lived experience of this transition, we'll develop a sense of what to expect and how to prepare for this time in our lives. In the postmenopausal years, we'll explore the grandmother hypothesis and find out what orcas and hunter-gatherer grandmothers have in common, the history and current state of hormone replacement therapy, and how developing our physical and mental grit is essential for our cognitive health and may even allow us to become "superagers."

We can think of the seasons of life as an act of becoming, or of moving into our deep selves, guided by a body that is at once always changing, but still recognizable in the same way that a path you've walked a thousand times is shaped by the changing seasons, but always familiar. What we do and do not pay attention to shapes our reality. That is, what we notice, observe, revisit, listen to, and tune in to changes the lens through which we interpret and understand the world and ourselves in it.

We can't always avoid getting pummeled by waves, but with better tools and knowledge, we can avoid getting stuck in a loop of crashing water and find relief in the sandy bottom that's just below the surface, waiting to support us. The way we navigate our environment, whether we're talking about open water or our overall health, is shaped by the tools and information we have at hand. This book is meant to provide you with enjoyable and accessible resources that empower you to find stability, relief, and joy in the experience of each cycle and season of your life.

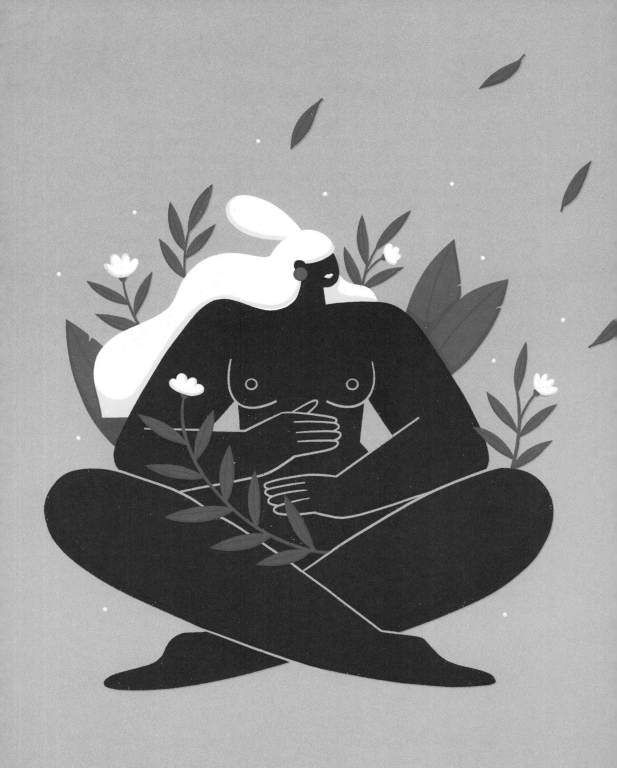

PART ONE

Reclaiming Your Cycle

These first few chapters act as the foundation to rebuild our perception of the menstrual cycle through a better understanding of our hormones, history, and health. This is the why and the how before we dive deeper into the details of each cycle's phase in the second part of the book.

Let's get one thing straight: this is not about romanticizing the menstrual cycle. Instead, we are acknowledging that the menstrual cycle is both biologically normal and, as the human rights activist, researcher, professor, and coeditor of *The Palgrave Handbook of Critical Menstruation Studies* Dr. Inga Winkler writes, fundamental because it "unites the personal and political, the intimate and the public, and the physiological and the socio-cultural." It is crucial to understand that we all experience our cycles differently and our experience is shaped by our unique contexts. The goal of Part One is to reclaim your cycle—what it means for you, how you experience it, and the story you tell yourself about your body. Valuing your menstrual cycle as a vital sign of health and understanding how it works hold great power. This power is about ownership and connection to your body; it's about knowing that your body is not broken or shameful, but that it is instead immensely adaptable and capable—and so are you.

Your Cycle Matters

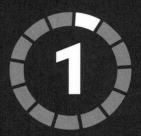

Before I ever got my period, my mom told me about the bleeding and showed me pads, tampons, and the paper in the tampon box with instructions for use in case you forgot. I was twelve years old and quietly confounded as she calmly told me about, what seemed to her, a normal and casual fact of life. I remember thinking, *Okay, this thing is going to happen, but why do we have to bleed at all and why does it happen every month?*

Me, You, and the Elephant Shrew

It would be about twenty years before I realized I was asking a hotly debated question that scientists have been trying to answer for a long time: why do humans with a uterus menstruate? The monthly shedding and regeneration of the endometrium—the innermost lining of the uterus—is rare among female mammals. Besides higher primates (think apes), bats, and elephant shrews, we're mostly alone in the animal kingdom when it comes to the way our bodies cyclically prepare for reproduction. To get to the heart of why we have a monthly menstrual cycle, it helps to think like an evolutionary biologist. Biologists study the process of life and living organisms; evolutionary biologists are interested in the patterns of life and how (and why) they change over time.

Thinking this way isn't perfect (there's plenty of sexist and racist evolutionary biologists scattered throughout human history), but it can help cut through cultural stories that reinforce negative menstruation stigmas and taboos. Historically, not all cultures considered menstruation taboo, but popular texts—think the Bible and other holy scriptures—advise people to avoid a menstruating woman because she is "unclean" and dirties everything she touches. In her article about the historical roots of menstrual stigmas, researcher and former science and education lead at Clue app Anna Druet writes that while menstrual taboos are common among diverse people and geographies, scholars don't agree about why these narratives surrounding menstruation were created. One theory, she writes, is that "menstrual taboos are at the center of the origins of patriarchy." This theory has two basic parts. First, in traditional, prehistoric hunter-gatherer cultures, women may have created their own menstrual taboo as a time when their bodies couldn't be touched, which gave them a powerful way to gain body autonomy. The next part of the theory is that this autonomy-generating menstrual taboo transformed from a practice that benefited females to one that did not.

Professor Chris Knight, the social anthropologist who developed this theory in his classic work *Blood Relations: Menstruation and the Origins of Culture*, argues that women created culture and that by limiting sexual contact during menstruation, they were able to collectively demand respect based on the sacredness of the body. A shift occurred when men started practicing ritualized bleeding and menstrual huts, where women traditionally gathered to menstruate, became men's territory for these bleeding rituals, which allowed men to co-opt the bleeding power of women. Women's ability to menstruate and give birth to children became associated with mystery and danger in many cultural myths, and so it was required for them to isolate during these reproductive events so that those forces could be controlled and suppressed. Knight writes that these early patriarchal cultures feared that "women's 'flows' might—in the absence of rules of seclusion or isolation—begin to synchronize, to connect up in a collective 'rhythm' or 'dance' over which men would have no control." He believes this change is the basis of the world's patriarchal religions.

This theory is appealing because it fits neatly into an idealized story of prehistoric matriarchal cultures where menstruation signaled empowerment. It has also been contested and debated because so much of the theory depends on menstrual cycle synchronization—both with other menstruators and the moon. This synchrony is not supported by recent research, though, anecdotally, many people who menstruate do experience a lunar connection and rhythm to their cycles. However, what Knight offers in his classic work (which, by the way, is about five hundred pages long), is a deep insight into the relationship between the stories our collective culture tells about menstruation and how those stories affect how people who menstruate are treated. Stories matter because they shape culture, and culture is the spoken and unspoken system we all live under and abide by.

ESSENTIALISM, GENDER, AND EVOLUTIONARY BIOLOGY

Most of us know that Charles Darwin developed the theory of natural selection in his breakthrough work *On the Origin of Species* published in 1859. But few of us think about how scientists explained evolution and the natural world pre-Darwin. For centuries before Darwin, scholars understood the concept of evolution, but not the mechanism, and science historians have pointed to one major obstacle that prevented these scholars from discovering the theory of natural selection: essentialism.

Pre-Darwin scholars believed that evolution occurred when a species' underlying essence was passed to the next generation, also described as the "transformational" theory of evolution. In contrast, Darwin formulated a "variational" theory of evolution; he recognized that variation within species was the primary mechanism of evolution. Despite Darwin's scientific findings, a 2008 study published in *Cognitive Science* found that most people have what the authors call an "essentialist bias"—they think of a species as a homogenous group with an underlying essence (pre-Darwin) instead of as a collection of unique individuals with intergroup variability (post-Darwin).

What we can learn from this research is that even if we understand and accept the theory of evolution, we may have a bias toward essentialism that prevents us from acknowledging and understanding the diversity and variability inherent to species. When applied to humans, essentialism is the idea that we have an innate nature that makes us who we are. Gender *essentialism* suggests that people have immutable, underlying maleness or femaleness that grants them specific masculine and feminine qualities. There are many problems with essentialism, especially when ideologies assert that human rights are tied to body parts as trans exclusionary radical feminists (TERFs) do. This group is especially dedicated to binary gender essentialism, which is harmful to people of all genders and especially oppressive and dangerous for nonbinary and transgender people.

Nonessentialism, on the other hand, acknowledges our differences and diversity, that each of us is unique and exists in unique cultural and environmental settings. Viewing the menstrual cycle as an experience that is innate to women and thus underlies the very definition and nature of "woman" is an essentialist view. We all experience our cycles, gender, and sex in unique and different ways. Darwin and other post-Darwin biologists recognized that a species' essence is not homogenous or fixed and this is the key to understanding natural selection—the very process that underlies our evolution as a species.

The power in thinking like an evolutionary biologist is that the perspective creates a different kind of story, which has the potential to generate a more equitable and egalitarian culture. Instead of thinking of menstrual blood as an unclean curse that proves we are uniquely mysterious and dangerous, thinking like an evolutionary biologist encourages us to ask the important questions: why did we evolve to have a menstrual cycle and what reproductive advantage does it give us?

There is growing evidence that people who menstruate abide by a cyclic reproductive rhythm because our collective uteri are "choosy." Meaning, my uterus and your uterus care about what happens inside them and have taken some steps over the last few million years to promote successful reproduction while also keeping people who menstruate and grow babies alive. The uterus evolved to be selective about the tiny organism—known as an embryo—that results when a sperm and egg unite because babies, even from their earliest, tiniest form, are uniquely invasive and costly for the body. If we experience pregnancy, babies implant in our uterus, tap into our blood supply, and get bigger and stronger by accumulating nutrition from our bodies for about forty weeks. Then we have to give birth and take care of the baby for years.

While we often think of pregnancy as a symbiotic relationship between a pregnant person's body and their baby, pregnancy is actually a conflict of competing genetic interests. Our basic, evolutionary drives are survival and reproduction. The more the fetus extracts from our bodies in the form of nutrition, the more likely it is to survive and reproduce. This is good for the fetus, but not great for us. If the fetus extracts too much from our bodies, it threatens our ability to survive and reproduce again. This conundrum, when the fetus and our body are attempting to maximize survivability and reproductive potential, is known as the *maternal-fetal genetic conflict*. To navigate this conflict, evolution and the process of natural selection shaped the relationship between the pregnant body and fetus so that the fetus could extract what it needed while the pregnant body put up some protections against total invasion and screened the embryos for their quality before investing in them for the long run.

Enter the menstrual cycle. While our menstrual cycles are often reduced to the bleeding phase and considered a monthly annoyance, an inconvenience, or worse, what we're actually talking about is a physiologic rhythm that is essential for life and orchestrated by our complex and interacting hormones. It is profoundly important to understand our cycles so that we can understand our overall health. By learning about our cycles, we learn about where we came from, how we got this way, how our bodies work, and how to support them.

Cycle Basics

Let's briefly review the physiology of the menstrual cycle, which we can think of as a monthly cycle of changes to the ovaries and endometrium (the uterine lining) that prepares the body for pregnancy through ovulation and ends with shedding the inner layer of the endometrium if pregnancy doesn't happen. The first day we have our period is considered day one of our cycle. The first phase of the cycle, from the beginning of menstruation to right before ovulation, is called the follicular phase. This phase is ruled by the hormone estrogen, which responds to another hormone, follicle stimulating hormone (FSH), which is released from the pituitary gland in the brain. FSH signals the ovaries to release estrogen, estrogen promotes endometrial layer growth and thickening and tells our cervical mucus to become friendly to sperm, and throughout this phase, one egg gets ready to burst out of the ovary. This bursting moment is the second phase of the menstrual cycle called ovulation, and it's triggered by another pituitary hormone, luteinizing hormone (LH). After ovulation, we enter the third phase of the cycle known as the luteal phase when progesterone is the dominant hormone, and it signals the pituitary to stop releasing FSH and LH. Progesterone focuses on increasing blood supply to the endometrium and decreasing endometrial thickness to create an environment that is friendly to a potential embryo looking for a warm place to implant and grow for the next forty weeks. In the absence of an embryo, the endometrial layer isn't maintained and is shed during menstruation, which is the fourth and final phase of the cycle.

What's special about the menstrual cycle is that it allows the endometrium to prepare for pregnancy without cues from an embryo and sheds this inner lining when pregnancy doesn't occur. This process is known as spontaneous decidualization. "Spontaneous," because, unlike many other mammals, our body is in charge of regenerating the inner lining instead of receiving cues from an embryo to develop. "Decidualization" refers to the process of preparing for pregnancy through cellular changes in the uterus. In some other mammals, embryonic cues tell the uterus to get ready for pregnancy. The embryo arrives and signals, "I'm here. Make this uterus comfortable!" The animal's body responds by building up the uterine lining. In our human bodies, even when there isn't a hopeful embryo hanging around, our hormones and immune system tell our bodies to prepare the endometrium to screen embryos if, by chance, one comes along. The idea behind this is simple: in other mammals, the embryo is in control; in our bodies, we are in charge.

The Menstrual Cycle

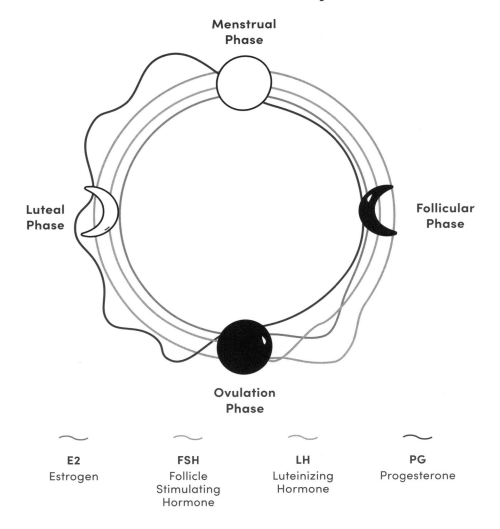

Menstrual Phase

Luteal Phase

Follicular Phase

Ovulation Phase

E2
Estrogen

FSH
Follicle Stimulating Hormone

LH
Luteinizing Hormone

PG
Progesterone

Menstrual phase: Estrogen and progesterone levels drop, triggering menstruation—the shedding of the uterine lining.

Follicular phase: Includes the first day of the period and ovulation. Rising estrogen levels causes the uterine lining to rebuild after menstruation.

Ovulation phase: The egg is released from the ovary after a spike in estrogen and luteinizing hormone.

Luteal phase: From ovulation until the beginning of bleeding, the uterine lining prepares either for pregnancy or shedding. The corpus luteum, formed after ovulation, secretes estrogen and progesterone during this phase.

Spontaneous decidualization also allows the body to sense the quality of the embryo when it implants. Because human embryos have a high rate of chromosomal abnormalities, spontaneous decidualization limits the investment in embryos that are unlikely to survive but increases the chance of reproductive success for quality embryos.

On average, throughout a lifetime, the endometrium cyclically sheds and regenerates around 400 to 450 times (there is, of course, great variation depending on the number of pregnancies, breastfeeding, and use of hormonal birth control). This ebb and flow maximizes reproductive success *and* survivability by allowing the uterus to be selective about the embryo it allows to implant during a narrow window of receptivity, also known as the *fertile* window. The highest chance of pregnancy is during the fertile window—five days before and on ovulation day. It's possible to get pregnant while on your period, or right after bleeding, especially if your cycles are twenty-one days long, but the chances of conceiving during this time are very low. And twenty-four hours after ovulation, the chances of conception are slim to none. By limiting the time when we can become pregnant, the menstrual cycle acts as an evolutionary strategy.

A Vital Sign

The menstrual cycle is considered the fifth vital sign that is just as important to assess and pay attention to as blood pressure, pulse, temperature, and respiratory rate. Vital signs give us some key information. First, they help tell us if there is an acute medical issue. Second, they inform us about the severity of disease or disorder in the body and how well the body is responding to physiological and emotional stress. Finally, they can indicate the presence of chronic diseases.

We understand this well when it comes to something like blood pressure. A single high blood pressure reading tells us that the body is responding to a stressor, but we don't know if the stressor is a singular event or a chronic disease-state. We have to monitor blood pressure over time to know if we're dealing with hypertension. Similarly, if you choose to pay attention to your menstrual cycles, you may gather valuable data about how your body is responding to your lifestyle in general including your diet, sleep patterns, exercise, and stress levels.

That said, if you are not experiencing a menstrual cycle with ovulation because of the use of hormonal contraceptives or gender-affirming hormone therapy, this doesn't imply that you are unhealthy. There are many strong opinions about whether menstrual cycles are even needed. On one side of this argument, people argue that not having a menstrual cycle is biologically wrong and leads to myriad health problems. On the other side of this argument, people argue that there is no medical reason to have a period and there is no shame or problem with tweaking our biology—especially when bleeding is painful. The only argument I buy into wholeheartedly is that the decision about experiencing a menstrual cycle, or blocking it with hormones, is a deeply personal one that you get to make as an individual.

Menstrual cycles can't be reduced to a singular measurement; they exist along a continuum with each phase giving us different information, or biomarkers, that help us understand our biology in real time. These biomarkers include physical signs such as cervical mucus patterns, cycle length, and cycle duration. We also have access to subtler signs of our health, like our energy levels and emotional state. As important as these physical and subtle indications of our cyclic health are to learn and understand, we are generally not taught to pay attention to these signs. In the United States, the cultural focus—including what is taught in health classes—is on the bleeding phase. There is an emphasis on the scientific explanation of the menstrual cycle, which leaves out the experience of the cycle, even though both the science and experience of the menstrual cycle are essential and offer vital information.

The medical approach to menstrual health tends to focus on regulating bleeding without paying as much attention to ovulation (unless we're trying to conceive) or other phases of the cycle. Ovulation, more than menstruation, allows us to interpret and understand our health during our reproductive years. This is because ovulation is a carefully orchestrated physiological event, and when we ovulate monthly, we're getting a signal that the glands and organs that make hormones in the body are functioning. If, on the other hand, we're not ovulating (and not preventing ovulation with medication like hormonal contraceptives or gender-affirming hormone therapy), we're getting information that something might be disrupting this system such as our lifestyle, diet, stress, or underlying conditions. When we only look at the bleeding phase of the cycle, it's like we're reading the conclusion to the story, but skipping over the good parts, ignoring the climax (ovulation), and missing some crucial details that allow the whole thing to make sense. Often, one of the first signs of an underlying health problem is a disruption in normal ovulation, followed by irregular cycles. Without understanding ovulation and the biomarkers that tell us we're ovulating, we miss out on the opportunity to notice abnormalities in our cycles and address them.

The menstrual cycle is like a story that gives us more information when we pay attention. Growing our understanding of this story improves our body literacy, which is the ability to understand and appreciate the body as a whole integrated system. Illiteracy, in all forms, whether we're talking about not being able to understand books or our own bodies, places decision-making power in the hands of those who have access to this information instead of those who are affected by the decisions.

Menstruation, as the authors write in *The Palgrave Handbook of Critical Menstruation Studies*, has been used by those who have power to impose conformity or uphold stigmas or worse on those who menstruate. The authors propose shifting this power back into the hands of those who menstruate by thinking about menstruation from a human rights perspective. Dignity and individual agency are central to human rights. Every person who menstruates deserves to both understand their body and exercise their agency.

Body literacy—gaining self-knowledge that leads to informed decision-making about health—paves the way for embodiment, which is the sense of being fully in our bodies and fully connected to ourselves through our senses. Part of body literacy, and thus embodiment, is learning how to pay attention to our bodily sensations. In the next chapter, we'll look at the history and impact of the tiny chemicals that majorly affect our bodily sensations: hormones.

The Naming of *Elixir Vitae*

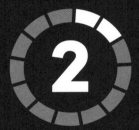

For scientists, discovering the endocrine glands and the hormones they produce was like finding magic in the body; the glands were the wands and the magic was these tiny chemicals that affected every organ system. The field of endocrinology—the study of the organs and glands that secrete hormones—is so vast, it spans both our physiology and psychology. Our hormones affect who we are, how we behave, our immune function and stress response, who we want to have sex with and if we want to have sex, metabolism, growth, sleep cycles, pregnancy, birthing, lactation, and parenting. Hormone shifts in our bodies shape the major phases of our life including puberty, our reproductive years, and the transition into menopause.

The discovery of hormones is an odd tale that combines some bizarre experiments with a bit of quackery. For example, ancient alchemists concocted "elixir vitae"—a fountain of youth—out of mashed-up animal testicles and ovaries. These elixirs were meant to fix a laundry list of ailments including low libido and aging. In 1889, at the age of seventy-two, the famous neurologist and professor of medicine at the Collège de France, Charles-Édouard Brown-Séquard, reported that he experienced incredible rejuvenation and improvements in his strength, ability to concentrate, and stamina after injecting himself with a mix of semen, juices from the testicles of dogs or guinea pigs, and blood from testicular veins.

Of course, Séquard and other scientists didn't use the terminology of "hormone" or "endocrinology." Experiments with sex organ elixirs occurred long before the word *hormone* was coined in 1905 by two British scientists and before the field of endocrinology existed. Until the early 1900s, scientists believed that signals traveled in the body solely via nerves, but the nervous system and endocrine system use different forms of communication to relay signals. The nervous system uses neural transmission, which sends certain messages along nerve tracts, while the endocrine system uses hormonal communication, which travels via our blood or circulatory system. If nerves are the telephone calls of the body sending their information via electrical signaling across synapses, hormones are like letters that get written in endocrine glands and delivered by our blood to specific target cells. Or you can think of hormones like your own inner Wi-Fi, as the medical writer Dr. Randi Hutter Epstein describes them. This form of communication, where tiny packets of chemicals create huge impacts on our organ systems and functioning, changed the way scientists thought about the body.

Instead of looking for microscopic nerve fibers connecting the organs, scientists found that specific glands in the body synthesized hormones and sent them off into the bloodstream, where they were able to bind to cells via specialized receptors at distant locations. Once hormones bind to their receptor sites, they initiate a cascade of cellular processes that end up modifying our physiology and/or behavior. The process of binding to receptors amplifies the cellular response, which is why extremely low concentrations of hormones can have a huge biological impact. The location of receptors shows us where the hormone is biologically active. This last bit is especially important, and it explains why our sex hormones have such broad, body-wide influences. Sex hormone receptors are located throughout the entire brain and body. They are in specialized brain cells, called glial cells, within our neurons, bones, immune cells, livers, and reproductive organs—the uterus, breasts, and gonads, either ovaries or testes.

Like most functions in the body, the brain coordinates and regulates the synthesis and release of our sex hormones through a communication pathway known as the HPO (hypothalamic-pituitary-ovarian) axis. Before puberty, this axis is rather quiet and our circulating levels of sex hormones are low as a result. Then comes the surge. During puberty, the HPO axis lights up, increasing its activity and initiating a cascade of physiological events. The action starts with the hypothalamus. This almond-sized structure is only about 0.4 percent of our total brain volume, but it has some big jobs, including the maintenance of physiological homeostasis and the management of reproductive function. The hypothalamus is responsible for sending out pulses of hormones that trigger the eggs in our ovaries to develop, and along with another hormone-secreting gland in the brain—the pituitary—it controls the menstrual cycle.

Meet Your Sex Hormones

In the late 1920s, two American researchers, Edward Doisy and Edgar Allen, started collecting urine from pregnant women. They did this unceremonious task because they were interested in an active substance secreted by the ovaries and found it plentiful in urine. They were looking to purify and isolate estrogen, which was assumed to be the female sex hormone, the hormone that made women more feminine and distinguished them from men, who had their own manly hormones.

While human urine samples provided scientists insight into estrogen, much of our understanding of the sex hormones was gained through animal research. Pigs, cattle, horses, and sheep all played a starring role in scientists' unique, and often gross, research methods. And so, it was by studying horse urine in the 1930s that scientists discovered estrogen was present in both mares and stallions. In fact, the amount of estrogen was higher in the urine of stallions. This finding stunned scientists and disrupted everything researchers understood and believed about sex hormones.

Up until this point, female and male sex hormones were used not only to describe biology but also behavior. Women's sex hormones were supposed to make them good wives and mothers—and if they stepped outside of these roles, it was because their female hormones were out of balance. The view that sex is binary, and that gender is oppositional (men versus women) is how the modern Western world, until very recently, understood and explained human biology. Unsurprisingly, the scientists studying hormones during this time were almost exclusively male and subscribed to the idea of biological determinism, which is the belief that human behavior is innate and determined by factors like genes, hormones, or brain size (versus factors like culture and geography). One of the obvious and massive repercussions of biological determinism is the belief that men are the natural, default sex and are thus physically and mentally superior to women. To be clear, biological determinism isn't based on science; it's a sexist ideology that manipulates the language of science to marginalize others, generally those are who not white cis men.

When scientists found that both mares and stallions, and subsequently humans, naturally have both "female" and "male" sex hormones, they had to reckon with the reality that, by their own definition, male and female weren't opposites. The ensuing gender bewilderment was later labeled an "epoch of confusion" by the physiologist Herbert Evans. The discovery that estrogen, progesterone, and testosterone were present in all people challenged the scientific and cultural understanding of what it meant to be a man or a woman. The discovery of hormones slowly opened the door to a wider understanding of sex and gender. Research shows that gender, which can be explained in many ways including personality traits, behaviors, and sexual attitude; and sex, a person's biological makeup composed of hormones, sexual characteristics, and chromosomes, are what one paper describes as "dimensional" rather than "taxonomic," which is the language scientists use to form two distinct categories. In other words, our biology is not binary.

Testosterone and estrogen are not only simultaneously present in all human bodies, but they are also related. If a person has testes, these organs produce testosterone. If the gonads present in the body are ovaries, these organs (along with the adrenal cortex and peripheral tissues) also produce testosterone, just in smaller amounts. Estrogen is formed when a special enzyme called aromatase converts testosterone into estrogen. Progesterone, another stereotypically "female" hormone that is sometimes called the "pregnancy hormone," was isolated and purified by scientists from the corpus luteum of female rabbits five years after estrogen was isolated and purified from urine. Like estrogen, higher quantities of progesterone are found in ovary-containing bodies, but it is also found in testes-containing bodies.

Hormones act throughout our brains and bodies, influencing our moods, behaviors, and physiology. The proportions of our sex hormones—testosterone, estrogen, and progesterone—determine the external and internal differences between people. To oversimplify it: all people are made using the same ingredients, but our bodies each follow a different recipe. While this metaphor applies all the way down to the level of our DNA, for hormones, where they are produced, the amount of them in our blood, and how they interact with different systems and organs affect how we look and how our bodies function.

In the first weeks of fetal development, we all look the same. Our bodies unfurl and sprout limb buds and the brain develops into a more complicated structure. The gonads, urged by genetics and hormones, undergo a complex transformation. Until sexual differentiation begins, a developing embryo has no hormonal or anatomic sex, just a genetic code (for example XX or XY). For the first five to six weeks of gestation, only the X gene expresses in both genetic codes. This X expression is often simplified into the idea that all humans start off as females, but the X is neither male nor female, meaning it's more accurate to say all humans start off with undeveloped and undifferentiated gonads. After five to six weeks of gestation, the gonads may differentiate into testes or ovaries while the external genitalia morph into a penis or vagina, or the external genitalia may be ambiguous as they are in some cases of intersexuality.

In her book *Aroused: The History of Hormones and How They Control Just About Everything*, Randi Hutter Epstein wrote about the complicated process of sexual differentiation and how hormones determine whether we develop testes, ovaries, or if we are intersex. Of this complicated process that requires precise timing and doses of hormones and genetic signaling, she wrote, "It's a wonder that any of us are born within the so-called conventional zone." The science of hormones encourages us to think of sex, identity, and gender along a spectrum and reminds us that diversity, rather than uniformity, is the rule of nature.

Those of us who experience a menstrual cycle do so because hormones produced by the hypothalamus, pituitary, and ovaries interact and tell our bodies to do different things at different times of the month. Our predominant sex hormones are estrogen and progesterone. Learning about these hormones teaches us that the whole body—not just our reproductive system—is affected by these (and many other) hormones. The next two sections cover these hormones and some of their basic body-wide effects.

HORMONE "BALANCE"?

Despite the numerous claims that a specific food, supplement, cleanse, herb, or other product will "balance" your hormones, the idea that hormones are either in or out of balance is imprecise. We tend to use the phrase "hormone imbalance" as a catchall description for feeling lousy or off, but it is not a medical diagnosis. The thing about hormones is that they are incredibly complex and there are more than fifty different hormones involved in our health. Hormones interact, fluctuate, and affect multiple organs and body systems. If you have symptoms that are typically labeled under the blanket phrase "hormone imbalance" including weight gain, PMS, fatigue, sleep issues, skin and hair changes, and anxiety or other mood changes, it's important to dig into the root cause, which is not always our hormones. A few examples of real hormonal disorders include hypothyroidism; polycystic ovarian syndrome (PCOS), when a person experiences irregular and/or anovulatory menstrual cycles (cycles without ovulation) and produces abnormally high androgen (testosterone-related) hormones; and hypothalamic amenorrhea (absent menstruation), when anorexia (lack or loss of appetite) or extreme exercise or weight loss results in the hypothalamus failing to signal ovulation.

Any supplement, product, or cleanse that promises to balance, detox, or reset your hormones should be met with skepticism. For the most part, our overall health, including our hormonal health, comes back to lifestyle and includes getting enough rest, reducing and managing stress, moving your body often, eating healthy food, and avoiding processed food, alcohol, and smoking. There is no quick fix or secret ingredient or special product you can buy to magically fix your hormones; there's just the day in, day out choices you make that help shape your health throughout your lifespan.

Estrogen

We can think of estrogen as a master regulator, coordinating complex signaling across genes, cells, and organs. At the onset of puberty, estrogen plays a role in the physical maturation of the breasts, ovaries, vagina, and uterus and stimulates the production of cervical mucus each month, which increases thirtyfold from the beginning of menses until ovulation.

Estrogen regulates genital blood flow, vaginal lubrication, and thickness and flexibility in the vaginal and urethral tissues. Along with the vagina, clitoris, and vulva, the pelvic floor, bladder, and urethra all contain receptors for estrogen, which gives these structures the strength and suppleness required for normal bladder, bowel, and sexual function.

Our immune function and the microorganisms that inhabit our bodies are also influenced and mediated by estrogen. In the vaginal microbiome, estrogen plays a key role in promoting a *Lactobacillus*-dominated environment. A healthy vaginal microbiome rich in *Lacto* offers greater protection against infections, such as sexually transmitted infections, by improving the immunological barriers of the cells lining the vagina.

In the musculoskeletal system, estrogen increases the collagen content of connective tissue and improves muscle strength and mass. Our hair growth is affected by estrogen, which explains why armpit and pubic hair begin growing during puberty and why plummeting estrogen levels postpartum can result in hair loss. Our skin—its collagen content, thickness, moisture, pigmentation, and overall appearance—is influenced by estrogen and changes throughout the month and over our lifetimes.

While we think of estrogen predominately as a reproductive hormone, it majorly affects how our brains develop and age. Estrogen is neuroprotective and studies find that it has an impact on regulatory functions and processes such as sexual behavior, appetite and eating behaviors, body temperature, anxiety, and cognition. Because estrogen levels peak when we're most fertile and we have receptors throughout our brain and body, researchers have spent decades debating whether our bodies signal our fertility status to potential mates via our behavior, appearance, and physiological cues.

What we can learn from this brief review of estrogen and its many effects within the body is that this hormone is so much more than a "female" sex hormone. It has far-reaching impacts on essential and basic functions and teaches us that we can't reduce our sex hormones to just sex.

THE FOUR ESTROGENS

Estrogens—that's right, there's more than one!—are a group of chemically similar steroid hormones. The three most common estrogens are estrone (E1—dominates during menopause), estradiol (E2—dominates during our nonpregnant reproductive years), and estriol (E3—dominates during pregnancy). The fourth, estetrol (E4), is a pregnancy-specific estrogen synthesized in the liver of a fetus. The most potent estrogen, and the one that people are generally referring to when they talk about estrogen, is estradiol. The action of each type of estrogen is mediated by estrogen receptors. When estrogen binds to an estrogen receptor, it triggers cellular changes. Estradiol is considered the strongest estrogen because it initiates substantially greater cellular changes and growth than the other estrogens, which are considered weak estrogens. Throughout this book, when you see "estrogen," this term is referring to estradiol unless otherwise noted.

Progesterone

While estrogen peaks right before ovulation and again during the mid-luteal phase (the second half of the cycle following ovulation and preceding menstruation), progesterone stays quiet during the first half of the cycle, building slowly and powerfully to become the dominant hormone during the luteal phase. Picture these two hormones as ocean waves with slightly different high tides that affect each other in a complex dance during the rhythm that is our cycles.

Progesterone acts as a priority-shifting chemical for our brains and bodies. While progesterone is associated with reduced sexual motivation, sex can still happen. Some research suggests that sexual motivation during the luteal phase exists to maintain strong bonds and relationships while other research fails to repeat these findings. Sex, like sex hormones, is dynamic and can't be reduced to a single variable. It's interwoven with everything else and varies from person to person as well.

Right before ovulation, progesterone levels start rising. The corpus luteum, a transient endocrine organ the luteal phase is named after, comes into existence following ovulation and secretes progesterone and estrogen. It grows stronger as the luteal phase progresses, but it only survives if human chorionic gonadotropin (hCG) is produced by a pregnancy. Without hCG, the corpus luteum stops functioning and breaks down. The resulting drop in both progesterone and estrogen triggers menstruation.

From the Latin *pro gestationem*, progesterone is most widely known for its vital role in maintaining pregnancy. Rising progesterone levels cause cervical mucus to become thick and impenetrable for sperm to pass through. Where estrogen signals the endometrium to thicken and grow, progesterone signals the endometrium to stop thickening and start secreting chemicals that increase blood flow and help stabilize and prepare it for potential embryo implantation. Progesterone's job is to shut down the ovaries so they don't release more eggs. By blocking ovulation, progesterone protects a potentially fertilized egg as it grows in the uterus. It sustains pregnancy both through its stabilizing effects on the endometrium and through its effects on our metabolism including how we use glucose and insulin, how and where body fat is stored, and through its effect on liver function, which is crucial for meeting the high demands of pregnancy. While progesterone is crucial for the development of a growing fetus, its impacts extend well beyond the contents of the uterus.

Like estrogen, progesterone is also neuroprotective. It is important for the development of our central nervous system and is involved in forming neural circuits and modulating memory, learning, and mood. It also acts as a smooth muscle relaxant, protects us from breast and uterine cancer, increases basal body temperature, and supports healthy sleep and thyroid function.

Endocrine Disruptors

Endocrine-disrupting chemicals are defined as chemicals or mixtures of chemicals that interfere with any aspect of hormone action and increase the risk of health problems such as reproductive and cognitive impairment, cancer, and obesity. The major groupings of these chemicals include industrial, agricultural, and residential sources that enter the body via food intake, inhalation, or direct contact. While endocrine-disrupting chemicals can interfere with any endocrine organ and impact many different hormones, their main targets include the endocrine axes that regulate thyroid, reproductive, immune function, and our stress response. Recent research also shows that these disruptors negatively affect metabolic health by increasing the number and size of fat cells, disrupting our satiety signaling, and reducing basal metabolic rate. Endocrine disruptors do their damage by mimicking or interfering with our endogenous (natural internal) hormones. They are like mini hackers, encouraging our endocrine glands to alter their hormonal production in ways that lead to issues throughout the body. From reproductive abnormalities to cancer or altered immune function and development, these disruptors pervasively interfere with the coordination and signaling that our endocrine system so tightly regulates.

Because endocrine-disrupting chemicals often mimic gonadal sex hormones, the reproductive system is especially vulnerable to disturbance. The ovaries and mammary tissues are finely tuned listeners and communicators. Because ovaries are such good listeners, they respond to tiny amounts of chemicals from our pituitary to initiate the process of egg development and ovulation. But they also listen to chemicals like bisphenol-A (BPA), which lines many food and drink containers. Exposure to BPA during our reproductive years affects egg quality and size and compromises embryo implantation, among other ill health effects. The impact of endocrine-disrupting chemicals is complicated because factors like age, life stage, sex, timing, and dose of exposure determine the effect. Basically, if we're exposed to higher levels of these chemicals at a younger age, the risk of negative health effects is generally greater.

These chemicals don't just disrupt our internal environment; they interfere with the health of our entire ecosystem—and the effects aren't trivial. Moreover, we do not all equally bear this burden: low-income populations as well as Latinx, Black, and other communities of color in the United States face significantly higher exposure to multiple endocrine-disrupting chemicals and therefore increased rates of metabolic disorders. This is an example of the intersection of racial, social, and environmental injustices. The disparity in exposure is rooted in systemic inequality and sociological forces such as reduced access to healthy food and increased exposure to toxic chemicals in low-income neighborhoods.

Improving environmental health is crucial to addressing these racial, income, geographic, and health inequities. Some actions we can take include advocating for equitable access to green space and the outdoors and recognizing that climate justice and social justice are inextricably intertwined. Major systemic changes are essential, corporations need to be held accountable for their pollution, and we need equal and expanded access to the fundamentals—healthy food, safe spaces, and nature—that nourish and sustain health.

The scope of environmental and social injustice are enormous, and good starting points that increase our understanding and compassion for this issue are awareness and humility. The table below lists everyday sources of endocrine disruptors and alternatives that reduce exposure to these chemicals. This table is not recommending that you immediately go out and buy all new, non-toxic products. Most of us don't have the time or money to do this. Instead, focus on small, attainable choices that benefit your health and the health of the environment—for example, swapping out single-use plastics for reusable products or replacing a nonstick pan with an inexpensive secondhand cast iron skillet. Additionally, if you don't have access to organic food, the best option is still to eat plentiful fruits and vegetables. It's not realistic to avoid everything that may potentially harm us, but it is realistic to increase our awareness and make small steps toward improving our health.

Endocrine Disruptors and Substitutes

TOXIN SOURCE	DANGEROUS CHEMICALS
Plastic products including plastic bottles, receipts, food packaging, plastic toys, PVC, plastic wrap	Bisphenol-A (BPA), phthalates, polychlorinated biphenyls (PCB), formaldehyde, heavy metals
Nonstick cookware, aluminum, and plastic kitchen utensils	Perfluoroalkyl and polyfluoroalkyl substances (PFAS), polytetrafluoroethylene (PTFE), perfluorooctanoate (PFOA), perfluorinated chemicals (PFCs)
Food grown with pesticides	Pesticides—triazines, pyrethroids, carbamates, organophosphates, organochlorides—herbicides, fungicides, rodenticides, glyphosate, perchlorate
Personal care and cleaning products: makeup, lotions, trash bags, shampoos, soaps, kitty litter, wipes, candles, laundry detergents, dryer sheets, skin, hair, and nail products, scented plug-ins, perfumes, etc.	Triclosan, artificial fragrances, phthalates
Furniture: couches, mattresses, chairs, baby car seats, electronics, foam cushions	Polybrominated diphenyl ethers (PBDE), PFAS
Fast fashion: cheap, disposable clothing	Herbicides, pesticides, phthalates, nonylphenol ethoxylates (NPEs), amines from azo dyes
Fish (swordfish, tilefish, king mackerel, shark, marlin), amalgam fillings and crowns, paint, some water pipes, toys, jewelry, occupations or hobbies that involve exposure	Lead and mercury

CHOOSE INSTEAD	(MORE) AFFORDABLE OPTIONS
Stainless steel, silicone, and glass (think mason jars) for food storage; BPA-free canned goods, reusable water bottles, beeswax wrap, ceramics free of lead, non-toxic reusable food storage bags, non-toxic baby and children's toys	Secondhand and thrift stores, big-box stores
Cast iron, stainless steel, and lead-free ceramic cookware; wood and stainless-steel utensils; porcelain, enamel, or ceramic-coated cookware and glass	Thrift stores for cast iron skillets. Any company selling non-toxic, affordable cookware.
Sustainably grown produce, pastured, free-range, and organic meats, wild fish and game, organic dairy, food grown using regenerative agriculture principles, wild-foraged foods	Farmers' markets, food delivery services such as Imperfect Foods and Farmbox, CSAs (community supported agriculture), community gardens, food banks, and pantries
Products free of added artificial fragrances and phthalates made by companies that disclose all of their ingredients. Check your personal care products on EWG Skin Deep Cosmetics Database. Clean with diluted vinegar and other non-toxic cleaners.	More brands are selling "green" products—but one of the best, and cheapest, housecleaning solutions is white vinegar diluted with water. With makeup and other personal care items, look for "fragrance, paraben, and phthalate-free."
Furniture and other goods made without flame retardants. If in doubt, call the manufacturer for information.	Reduce exposure by opening your windows, washing your hands, vacuuming often, mopping and dusting, and before buying anything new, check that it's made without flame retardants.
Organic, recycled, and natural fibers made by brands that focus on sustainability, fair conditions for workers, and environmental stewardship	Secondhand clothes that are 100 percent cotton or wool
Fish: Wild salmon, sardines, herring, anchovies, oysters, squid, skipjack tuna, sole, squid, scallops, cod, clams, black sea bass, freshwater trout, sole, shrimp	Canned fish like sardines and anchovies, on sale wild/fresh or frozen fish and seafood

Evolving Self-Knowledge

In a conversation with Krista Tippett, the philosopher Alain de Botton said that one of the narcissisms of our time is that we think we've arrived at the pinnacle of human knowledge. We think we're "latecomers to the party," he said, but "we're still at the very beginning of understanding ourselves as human, emotional creatures." When it comes to understanding the world and our bodies, we're very much just arriving at the party. Acknowledging the reality that we know very little curates a sense of humility, and maybe even awe. What we need, Botton says, is more compassion as we take baby steps toward understanding ourselves.

The history of hormones demonstrates that our ability to understand ourselves and our bodies exists in the wider context of current scientific and cultural norms—how we perceive who we are changes as we learn more and as our world changes. As much as we know, we will always also be defined by what we don't know. In this way, learning about the body is an ongoing and evolving process of self-knowledge. Our evolving understanding of self requires the ability to unlearn and relearn, a commitment to open-mindedness, and a willingness to move beyond a binary understanding of the world and our biology and toward a more nuanced and diverse understanding.

The Cycle &
The Brain

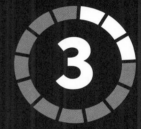

If you've ever been told you're acting "hormonal" when you're just expressing an opinion or been made to feel that you're not good at math, sports, or navigation because of your sex, you've experienced the effects of a myth that has persisted in our world for centuries. This is the myth of androcentrism, and it was invented by the patriarchy. Though there are many ways to historically trace the lineage of this type of thought, part of it came from science. Science is culturally significant, shaping everything from how we eat and exercise to our views about sexuality and education and who gets to participate in what. And, science is not immune to societal issues like institutionalized racism and sexism. In fact, when it comes to reproductive health and menstruation, there is no shortage of biased science. Since the beginning of our scientific journey to understand the human body, scientists (most of whom, of course, happen to be men) have treated the male body as the default. So women, and any other individuals who are not stereotypically cisgender males, are seen as biologically inferior to men. Part of the evidence scientists use to uphold this claim was, and still is to an extent, the menstrual cycle.

For example, during the late 1800s, the Harvard physician Edward H. Clarke wrote his popular and persuasive book, *Sex in Education; or a Fair Chance for the Girls*. In it, he argued that higher education was inappropriate for women because intensive study would divert energy from the uterus to the brain. He made this and many other claims about women's health based on "clinical observations" and "physiology." For example, he presented a case about a smart and anxious young girl who studied too hard at school—or as Clarke wrote, "just as boys do"—who developed painful periods. His assessment was that this was because school required her brain to work hard while nature required her reproductive system to function, and due to her "delicacy and weakness" as an American woman, her body was unable to physiologically multitask, so her menstrual health suffered. The brainpower required for education, he argued, defied physiological laws. He concluded that the pursuit of higher education would cause uteri to atrophy, menstrual cycles to become irregular, and women to become "irritable and infertile." Here was an educated, influential doctor and professor who preached that menstruation was debilitating and promoted the exclusion of people who menstruate from intellectual stimulation. Clarke's work combined personal theory with science and was considered cutting edge in the 1870s. The result was a sexist text that took the position of looking out for women's best interests when it was really denying their rights. Clarke's work and influence are a terrifying example of how the authority and perceived "truth" of science can be dangerous for the race or sex of anyone who is considered "other" and doesn't fit the status quo of nondisabled, white, cisgender male.

While we know now that menstruation doesn't prevent us from learning and intellectual engagement, you might be wondering if and how the menstrual cycle does affect cognition. A 2017 study published in *Frontiers in Behavioral Neuroscience* looked at cognition as it relates to the phases of the menstrual cycle. The researchers examined three aspects of cognition—working memory, cognitive bias, and the ability to pay attention to two things at once—and found that the levels of testosterone, estrogen, and progesterone had no impact on any of these functions. The study used a larger sample size compared to similar studies and, crucially, followed individuals across two consecutive menstrual cycles. By tracking cognitive effects over two cycles, the researchers were able to examine whether changes in cognition repeated. Analysis of the first menstrual cycle showed some effects in attention and cognitive bias, but these effects failed to repeat in the second menstrual cycle. This means that the study's authors couldn't make a meaningful or consistent association between hormone levels and the type of cognitive functioning the study measured.

This research offers a needed challenge to the scientific methodology used in recent papers linking cognitive functioning to hormone levels. Many studies that claim there is a link between cognition and hormone levels show poor evidence, small sample sizes, inflated effects, poor reproducibility, and a high degree of bias. This is the language scientists use to say that these studies are full of inconsistencies and need to be reexamined. Worse still, these dramatic findings often end up in the news, falsely linking cause and effect and embedding relationships into our cultural psyche that don't exist. Zooming in on the key issue, the researchers of the 2017 study questioned if cyclic sex hormone levels actually consistently affect cognitive functioning or whether other studies' "positive findings are spurious false-positives due to scientific fallacies and methodological biases."

We need science to reexamine assumptions from a different angle and question deeply held beliefs. Not surprisingly, when scientists themselves are more diverse (i.e., not all cis straight white guys), the types of questions that get asked and the way they are answered change too. For example, a review conducted by three women and published in *Brain Sciences* in 2020 found that studies examining the relationship between cognition and menstrual cycle phases haven't been able to consistently show that normal hormone fluctuations alter cognitive abilities. The authors suggested that perhaps the sex difference hypothesis is simply outdated. They also proposed the idea that our cognitive strategies, rather than abilities, change during different menstrual cycle phases. (More on this in the next section!)

I opened this chapter this way for a few reasons. First, there's a lot of information out there about how hormones and the menstrual cycle have an impact on our brains and bodies. Instead of accepting what we're told about ourselves as irrefutable facts, we can instead look at both science and anecdotal experiences with healthy skepticism and a willingness to reconsider, relearn, and perhaps unlearn what we hold as true. Second, and most important, the recognition that some of our deepest held beliefs and assumptions about ourselves may be influenced by decades of bias grants us the freedom to pause and ask, *Is this really true?* When we look at ourselves through a different lens, we might be surprised to find that from one cycle to the next, we dismantle some deeply held—yet spurious—myths about who we are and how our bodies and minds operate.

Sex Hormones, the Brain, and Behavioral Immunity

Our brains are not fixed, unchanging structures. They are highly plastic and able to adapt to our environment and experiences. Some research has found that estrogen and progesterone affect neural plasticity in regions of the brain that perceive and store memories. For a long time, we've understood, both through science and anecdotally, that emotional events tend to be remembered better than neutral events. These drama-filled moments, whether great or traumatic, tell our bodies to release adrenal hormones, which prompt our brains to store and consolidate these memories. This explains why I can't forget that time five years ago when my jeans split at the climbing gym when my now-husband was belaying me, while at the same time, I can't remember what I had for dinner last night.

Not only do we tend to remember emotionally heightened experiences better and in greater detail, how we process and store those memories is affected by the phase of our menstrual cycle. A 2019 review in *Frontiers in Neuroendocrinology* elaborated on the connection between ovarian hormones, memory, how fear is regulated in the brain, and post-traumatic stress disorder (PTSD)—which cisgender women are twice as likely as men to suffer from. After reviewing the available evidence, the authors found a consistent relationship between levels of estrogen, progesterone, and allopregnanolone and PTSD symptoms. Higher levels of these hormones are believed to confer resilience to PTSD (think during the mid-follicular and early luteal phase), while low levels put us at higher risk of PTSD symptoms (as in the late luteal and early follicular phase). The takeaway from this review is that how we respond to trauma, fearful experiences, and stressful situations is affected by fluctuating ovarian hormone levels across the menstrual cycle, and we may be at higher risk when those levels are lowest.

Our sex hormones may also influence how we perceive or recognize others' facial expressions and our reaction to negative stimuli. Researchers suspect that progesterone, or at least the higher ratio of progesterone in relationship to estrogen, is responsible for emotional processing changes. When progesterone starts to rise after ovulation, we tend to perceive fearful expressions as more intense, react faster to angry or sad situations, and pay more fearful attention to potentially dangerous creatures like snakes. Additionally, our disgust response can become more intense so that we are more repulsed by things or situations that gross us out or threaten us.

Research suggests that menstruating people are better at emotional recognition during the follicular phase and more tuned in to danger and other negative stimuli during the luteal phase. Though everyone's experience will differ from person to person and cycle to cycle, what this trend might mean is that we're more tailored toward social interaction during the follicular phase and more focused on protecting ourselves from social threats during the luteal phase.

One explanation for the change in emotional processing and brain reactivity throughout the month is that estrogen and progesterone affect how the immune system operates. Because our bodies can grow a new life-form, we need an intelligent and dynamic immune system. Our bodies must be able to attack whatever bug is threatening our health and also recognize that a fetus is not one of those bugs.

Just like our brain is plastic and changeable across our cycles, so too is our immune function. Immune cells are loaded with receptors for estrogen and progesterone, shifting between inflammatory and anti-inflammatory responses as the levels of each hormone change. When estrogen and progesterone increase after ovulation and there's a chance we might be pregnant, our immune response transitions to a more tolerant state by decreasing inflammatory responses. Not only does the body need to tolerate a potential embryo, but it also needs to screen embryos for their viability while protecting us from harmful pathogens. Here, we can connect immune function with cycle-mediated changes in perception and behavior. Progesterone's main job is to sustain pregnancy. It does this through specific physiological mechanisms, like cultivating an anti-inflammatory environment in the body as well as by modifying our behavior.

During the happy, carefree follicular phase, some research shows that people who menstruate tend to be more social and more sexually active. Then, progesterone acts like a behavioral prophylactic, increasing our sensitivity to threats and danger. Taken together, these effects are meant to decrease our exposure to disease when we are most vulnerable to infection. Therefore, the change in our emotional processing from the first to the second half of our cycles may act as an adaptive defense mechanism.

Jacobi versus Clarke

In 1876, three years after Clarke published *Sex in Education*, Mary Putnam Jacobi won the honorary Boylston Prize at Harvard Medical School for her paper, "The Question of Rest for Women During Menstruation." She was a trailblazer who received her first MD from the Woman's Medical College of Pennsylvania in Philadelphia and her second MD from the École de Médecine in Paris, where she was also the first woman admitted.

Like Clarke, Jacobi saw science as a conduit for political action. But, where Clarke aimed to build barriers to entry for women, Jacobi worked to dismantle gender-based obstacles that created a divided, hierarchal, and patriarchal society. In response to Clarke's work that reflected his biased personal theories, Jacobi's paper focused on analysis, charts, and data that examined cisgender women throughout their menstrual cycle. Among other analyses, she had her subjects perform muscle strength tests before, during, and after menstruation to demonstrate that menstruation didn't cause muscle weakness. She knew that sexism and biological determinism needed to be challenged with good science and strong women.

Her findings contradicted Clarke's theory that menstruating people who sought education would suffer physical depletion and sterility because of some supposed fragile constitution. She argued that when women were educated, physically active, and mentally engaged, they were actually healthier. Menstruation was not a disease-state that biologically weakened women. It did not require exemption and exclusion from society. As the historian Carla Bittel wrote in her biography of Jacobi, "social limitations, not biology, constrained women and threatened their health."

The world has changed since Clarke and Jacobi shared their opposing views on where menstruating people fit in the intellectual landscape. We can use our brains in whatever form we choose without worrying about compromising our fertility or enfeebling our physiology—which is far from fragile. But menstruation is still stigmatized, and people who menstruate still face social limitations. Studies still emerge that link abilities to biology, and many people—especially those on the margins—continue to face threats to their reproductive rights. As Jacobi demonstrated, menstruation is political. Better, more scientifically sound information changes how we understand the human body.

Eat, Move, (Self) Love

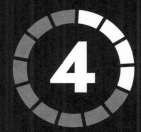

In ancient Greek, the word *diet* referred to a "mode of life" and encompassed food and drink, massages and baths, sun therapy, sleep, sexuality, habits, and exercise. Diet was an expansive description of lifestyle. I imagine the Greek meaning of the word *diet* as a large, idyllic platter that each essential part of life is served from. A warm drink and eggs for breakfast, a massage and a long walk in the sun for brunch, fish and vegetables for lunch, followed by a restoring nap. An afternoon tryst, a dip in the ocean followed by a bath, a fulfilling dinner, chocolate truffles, another evening walk, and finally a restful night of sleep. Even on days when work predominates, I like to think, *How can I improve my diet today?*

Though this expansive definition prevailed over two thousand years ago, nowadays, "diet" usually refers to eating as a path to weight loss. Diet no longer encapsulates a mode of life that promotes spiritual, physical, and emotional balance; it's focused on deprivation. Diet culture is obsessed with thinness and uses methods like calorie counting and restriction to enforce vanity-based ideals. The wellness industry, under the guise of improving health, promotes "clean eating"—just another way to sell weight-loss diets (think juice cleanses and elimination diets) that demonize certain foods like carbs, dairy, nightshades, and all forms of sugar. In her 2019 *New York Times* piece "Smash the Wellness Industry," Jessica Knoll says the wellness industry is a con that uses pseudoscience to trick smart women into fearing certain foods to improve their health. "But, at its core, 'wellness' is about weight loss," she writes. "It demonizes calorically dense and delicious foods, preserving a vicious fallacy: thin is healthy and healthy is thin."

It's worth reclaiming a broader definition of diet because of this vicious fallacy, and because food is more than just nutrients. Food is nourishment and pleasure; it connects us to our environment and to each other. The definition of diet has been narrowed down to food and then reduced again to isolated nutrients. This change is akin to a carrot being plucked from a garden where it existed with plants, animals, fungi, and bacteria. Now, in the hands of a human, the carrot becomes something singular, removed, and its essential "carrot-ness" is replaced by nutrient descriptors like beta-carotene, biotin, and vitamin K. Often, we treat our health like the carrot, removing ourselves from the complex ecosystem that makes us whole by renaming each separate part.

While the trend in nutrition science is to study singular nutrients, many studies show that whole foods, and especially combinations of whole foods, offer benefits beyond any singular nutrient. This is nature's way of reinforcing one of its most important and basic principles: diversity is essential. Ecologists have long understood that ecosystems rich in diverse species are substantially healthier and more productive than those where diversity is depleted. Diversity is the thread that ties together a community's health and resilience; the ecosystem within the body follows this same principle. The narrow list of foods that are considered healthy in the United States is a good example of a loss of diversity. The recipes in the second part of this book provide examples of the types of foods that help support overall health, but they are a sampling, not a comprehensive whole. Where you live, what grows locally and wildly, your culture and traditions—all these pieces make up the puzzle of what you eat. It is too reductive to say that we should all eat the same foods to benefit our health. We are all carrots growing in different gardens—maintaining and celebrating that diversity is essential.

Now that we've established that "diet" is a mode of life and diversity is fundamental to the health of every living thing, let's apply this balanced approach to blood sugar stability. Diabetes, the chronic metabolic disease that results from elevated blood sugar levels, is increasingly common in the United States. In 2020, the CDC's National Diabetes Statistics Report found that thirty-four million people are diabetic while over one hundred million people over the age of eighteen are prediabetic, meaning their blood sugar is high, but not high enough to be classified as diabetic. Prediabetes is associated with an increased risk of all-cause mortality and cardiovascular disease. What this means is that blood sugar levels matter for everyone, whether or not we carry a diabetes diagnosis. In the next sections, we'll look at how food, and blood sugar levels specifically, influence hormonal health, and then we'll talk about the other essential pieces of diet: movement and self-care.

Food: (Blood) Sugar and Sex (Hormones)

Glucose is a paradoxical molecule. On the one hand, it is critical for energy metabolism and life itself. But on the other, too much of it is potentially catastrophic for our health. To deal with this glucose conundrum, our bodies evolved mechanisms that help keep glucose levels within narrow physiological limits. Insulin is one of those mechanisms. This hormone stimulates glucose uptake into tissues and the liver, and it plays a key role in both carbohydrate and fat metabolism. One of its major, well-known jobs is to decrease blood glucose levels. When blood glucose levels are chronically high (hyperglycemia), our health suffers and the complications can include serious damage to nerve endings, blood vessels, eyes, kidneys, and the heart. In type 1 diabetes, hyperglycemia develops because cells in the pancreas called beta cells that produce and secrete insulin, and thereby regulate the amount of glucose in the blood, are damaged and destroyed by autoimmune dysfunction. Type 2 diabetes, on the other hand, develops when less insulin is produced by beta cells and the tissues in the body become less sensitive to insulin. The combination of not enough insulin and insulin resistance is a mismatch between how much insulin is available and how much the body needs to balance blood glucose levels. The result again is blood sugar levels that are too high and therefore disturb metabolic and overall health.

When the cells in the body stop responding to insulin—which is a complex process that includes genetics, metabolic, and environmental factors such as obesity, sedentarism, and unhealthy eating—insulin resistance develops and glucose isn't able to enter the cells. The body, attempting to maintain homeostasis, urges the beta cells to pump out more and more insulin. Higher levels of insulin are damaging to the blood vessels and contribute to body-wide health problems such as diabetes, high blood pressure, and heart disease.

When we eat too much sugar in the form of added sweeteners, refined carbohydrates, or excessive starchy foods, our bodies respond to the spike in our blood sugar by secreting a big dose of insulin. This insulin surge, among many other body-wide effects, reduces the amount of sex hormone binding globulin (SHBG), a protein made by the liver that helps control the amount of estrogen and testosterone in the body. Lower levels of SHBG lead to an increase in the release of estrogen and testosterone. The increase in these hormones is associated with increased body fat (which produces more estrogen), polycystic ovaries, acne, infertility, and uterine cancer.

While a diet heavy in processed foods and carbohydrates—especially of the refined, sugary, and high-glycemic variety—causes high blood glucose levels, certain foods (along with restful sleep, exercise, and other lifestyle habits) can help normalize and stabilize blood sugar. This is important because glycemic variability, meaning a blood sugar level that bounces around instead of staying at a stable level, is linked to an increased risk of cardiovascular disease and other complications in those with type 2 diabetes. Our blood sugar levels tend to bump up after sugar-heavy meals and this increase following meals is called postprandial hyperglycemia. The standard Western breakfast of processed foods, pastries, and cereal is a perfect setup for postprandial hyperglycemia.

Sex hormones also play a role in glucose homeostasis. Estrogen promotes insulin sensitivity (how your body responds to insulin) while progesterone may cause a decrease in insulin sensitivity. Some studies and anecdotal evidence find that, compared to the follicular phase, the luteal phase is associated with increased fasting blood sugar levels and postprandial hyperglycemia. Other studies fail to repeat this finding. The only way to know if you personally experience increased glycemic variability at different phases in your cycle is to take consistent measurements of your blood sugar and track what you eat. Most people who do not have a diagnosis of type 1 or type 2 diabetes don't track their blood sugar levels,

Support Healthy Blood Sugar Levels

Movement

Aerobic movement: walking, swimming, cycling

Resistance training: weightlifting, body weight movements (squats, pushups, climbing)

Move beyond exercise— build movement into your whole day

Whole Foods

Leafy greens and vegetables

Whole fruits

Whole grains

Reduce packaged and processed foods

Herbs, Teas, and Ferments

Cinnamon

Ginger

Turmeric

Green and Pu-erh tea

Apple cider vinegar

Sauerkraut, kimchi, lacto-fermented vegetables

Water

High-Quality Protein and Fats

Pasture-raised chicken and eggs

Wild game, fish and seafood

Grass-fed beef and lamb

Organic tempeh

Beans, legumes, nuts and seeds

Olive oil

Rest and Sleep

7–9 hours of sleep per night

Daily mindfulness practices: yoga, meditation, nature walks, baths, or journaling

Reduce screen time, especially before bedtime

Signs a Food Might Be Spiking Your Blood Sugar

Fatigue

Weight gain

Headaches

Trouble concentrating

Try adjusting or reducing total carbohydrate intake during meals and know that we are all different but if you're looking for data on the cyclicity of your metabolism and how food affects your blood sugar variability, a glucometer or continuous glucose monitor gives you access to this information.

Whether or not you are monitoring them, we can take steps to improve insulin sensitivity and lower blood glucose levels. The first step is to limit and reduce the intake of sugary foods, refined carbohydrates, juices, sugary drinks, and high-glycemic foods, especially in the morning when they appear to have the biggest impact on blood sugar. There is also evidence that eating protein- and fat-rich foods before ingesting carbohydrates, known in the literature as a "preload," improves glucose tolerance. There are also some other ingredients crucial to glucose metabolism, including vitamin D—which we get from the sun, supplementation, and foods such as oily fish, egg yolks, and fortified cereals—that impact glucose tolerance, insulin secretion, and insulin sensitivity. Some research suggests a deficiency is a potential risk factor for developing insulin resistance leading to Type-2 diabetes.

There is also a relationship between low vitamin D levels and menstrual disorders. In one study, cisgender women who did not meet the minimum recommended level of 30 ng/mL (nanograms per milliliter) of 25 (OH)D experienced five times the odds of menstrual cycle disorders compared to those who had sufficient levels. By the way, 25 (OH)D is the major circulating form of vitamin D in the body, and it is the only measurement that tells us whether we have sufficient levels. There is controversy about optimal vitamin D supplementation. The current recommended dietary allowance (RDA) of vitamin D for adults aged ninety to seventy years old is 600 IU/day with an upper limit of 4000 IU/day. Because vitamin D synthesis depends on so many factors, like where you live, your skin color, lifestyle, sun exposure, genetics, diet, and so on, for most people, it makes sense to supplement with sunshine (about fifteen minutes of midday sun exposure), vitamin D rich foods, and vitamin D_3. If possible, get your vitamin D levels drawn once a year so you know your baseline.

The recommendations for the general population when it comes to preventing type 2 diabetes and improving glucose metabolism are broad, and in some cases, medication is absolutely necessary. Our overall diet, eating patterns, and the amount and quality of food we eat matter. Crucially, focusing on whole foods offers greater benefits to our health. Certain foods and herbs like cinnamon, leafy greens, vinegar, green and Pu-erh tea, fermented foods, ginger and garlic, turmeric, oysters, and vitamin K_2 from foods like natto and chicken liver have some evidence behind them for improving our insulin response. Lifestyle habits like moving often (especially walking daily and resistance training) help improve insulin sensitivity. And, importantly, restful sleep, stress reduction practices like meditation, and positive social interactions and relationships all influence how our bodies respond to the food we eat and improve insulin sensitivity.

Movement: The Gym versus the Garden

Imagine you're in a gym. Exercise is available in familiar, culty forms like Peloton, Barre, SoulCycle, and CrossFit, along with kickboxing, yoga, HIIT, weightlifting, or if you're my friend's mom, extremely competitive pickleball. Next, imagine you're in the garden and there's not a $2,000 high-tech stationary bike in sight, but rather, the environment that surrounds you invites you to move. This might mean climbing a tree to pick an apple, foraging for a morel in the springtime, squatting to examine a freshly blossomed flower, crawling to play with your nephew, lifting a wheelbarrow full of soil, and walking anywhere and everywhere.

I love the gym and sometimes even enjoy dabbling in the pseudospiritual fitness cults that are so popular among millennials, but with two small children, my weightlifting and cardio often consist of picking up and carrying my kids and chasing after them. What happens when we expand the definition of exercise to include all kinds of movement is that we expand the ways we can live a healthy life. The movement recommendations in this book focus on cultivating an environment that invites you to move more. That might mean hanging a pull-up bar outside your bathroom, so you hang and swing after each bathroom trip, or doing something a little more radical like sitting on the floor during mealtimes so you're forced to practice greater mobility and strength each time you sit down. The idea behind this change in thinking is for you to break free from the idea that you need a gym to exercise and start to look at your surroundings as opportunities for movement. Not moving enough is directly tied to top diseases including obesity, diabetes, hypertension, cardiovascular disease, and cancer. Sedentarism also comes with a risk of mental health issues like depression, anxiety, and stress. As industrialized societies have moved further away from the movement-loaded lifestyles we used to live, our bodies have changed in response.

A study looking at hunter-gatherers' bones from seven thousand years ago found that compared to us modern *Homo sapiens*, our forager ancestors had more robust, stronger skeletons. The development and evolution of the human skeleton depends on frequent loading, also known as movement. The authors of the study, Dr. Timothy Ryan and Dr. Colin Shaw, wrote of their findings that "contemporary humans live in a cultural and technological milieu incompatible with our evolutionary adaptations." We are getting weaker, with higher rates of age-related bone loss, osteoporosis, and fractures because we don't move enough.

The standard takeaway from studies like Ryan and Shaw's is to exercise more. Do more strength and resistance training, try a virtual exercise program, get to the gym! These suggestions inform a change to part of our life, not a change to our way of life. The thing is, even if we add an hour of strength and resistance training to our exercise routine a few days a week, which is a great change, many of us with desk jobs spend the rest of the hours each day sitting down. Instead of thinking about adding exercise, we might consider subtracting the amount of time we spend not moving at all. Because we don't need to forage to survive, moving more consistently is challenging. Figuring out how to sit less is not a problem you can solve in a day. Rather, it is a daily practice that starts with a basic question, *How can I move more right now?* This might encourage a simple movement like taking a deep breath, reaching your arms up over your head and stretching, or switching from a chair to a yoga ball while you work.

Movement is also directly related to our reproductive and hormonal health. Muscle contractions help the uterine lining shed during menstruation and also move eggs and sperm along in the reproductive tract. Contractions of the uterus lead to childbirth. The endocrine organs are supported by skeletal muscles, which orient us to our environment through sensory receptors that tell us about our body position. Urinary and immune function, the cardiovascular system and breathing, digestion, and the nervous system—all of these systems rely on both skeletal and smooth muscle movements.

The tiny moving pieces of these systems, cells, also require movement to function. When we sit for too long, we compromise cellular functioning at the mechanical and chemical level. Sitting has an estrogenic effect on the body, meaning the more we sit, the higher our levels of estrogens, specifically estradiol and estrone. High blood levels of these two estrogens are linked to obesity (especially central obesity), inflammation, and estrogen-related cancers like breast cancer. The bottom line: sitting for hours every day is bad for us in every imaginable way.

The good news about moving more is that it's good for us in every way. People who move more and sit less experience decreased prevalence and lower intensity of the top PMS symptoms including pain with menstruation, breast pain, headaches, anxiety, depression, and irritability. There are several explanations for this reduction in the physical and psychological symptoms associated with PMS. Physical activity reduces the hormone prolactin in the late luteal phase, which can cause breast pain and swelling. The activity of renin, a hormone that affects the reabsorption of sodium and water, decreases with physical activity so we feel less bloated. Consistent and frequent movement improves venous blood return, which reduces discomfort in the stomach, pelvis, and back. Resting levels of norepinephrine decrease with regular physical activity, effectively reducing heart rate and blood pressure, which has an impact on both physical and psychological symptoms. An increase in brain endorphins and a decrease in adrenal cortisol help lessen anxiety and depression.

This is a short list of the hormonal benefits of moving more. As important as it is to move more, this doesn't necessarily boil down to exercising more; overexercising also has negative impacts on hormonal health. When we do too much repetitive movement, whether sitting too much or performing only one type of exercise every day, it's like only eating broccoli when we're trying to eat healthily. We need a more imaginative and diverse plate. In Parts Two and Three, you'll find ideas about how to increase both the amount and the diversity of movement in your life so that whether you're sitting and working at a desk or on your feet all day, you can increase your overall strength, balance, and comfort in your body.

Self-Care: Self-Preservation

If you look at a few hundred of the more than forty-eight million #selfcare posts on Instagram, you'll find such a wide range of things that you might wonder what self-care actually is. Weight-loss comparison photos, inspirational quotes, a few pictures of Keanu Reeves, skin care products, and many (*many*) glamorous selfies tie this loose concept together into a random amalgamation of, well, everything. And maybe this is kind of great—self-care is anything you want it to be. But there's also a problem here, especially as self-care has grown into a $450 billion industry (as of 2020) that often preys on our anxiety and insecurity by selling us ways to exert control and discipline on our bodies with expensive green juice and luxury skin care protocols.

There are alternatives to the product-centered, capitalistic industry of self-care. In her 1988 essay collection *A Burst of Light*, Audre Lorde famously wrote, "Caring for myself is not self-indulgence, it is self-preservation, and that is an act of political warfare" The concept of self-care as a political act has roots in the women's liberation and civil rights movements where women saw self-care as a reclamation of autonomy. The writer Aisha Harris wrote in her essay "A History of Self-Care" that "women and people of color viewed controlling their health as a corrective to the failures of a white, patriarchal medical system to properly tend their needs." We may also think of self-care as a way to preserve our capacity for connecting to and caring for others by first caring for ourselves—like putting on your own oxygen mask before placing one on your child. The writer and poet Angela Davis built on this idea when, in a 2016 interview with her sister Fania, she said, "Self-care and healing and attention to the body and the spiritual dimension—all of this is now a part of radical social justice struggles." Crucially, she explained that your interior life is connected to what happens in the world around you. So caring for yourself is an act of creating a better world.

Reclaiming the meaning of "self-care" is an act of choice, and it's a type of resistance. When we choose to turn away from what advertisements and commercial-based social media tell us we need, we can turn toward ourselves and pay attention to what we actually need. Ideally, self-care allows us to face the burdens of living without succumbing to the dangers of chronic stress. Stress, the kind that is persistent and long-term, comes from many different places. Racial and gender-based oppression and violence are types of extreme stressors that inform both Davis and Lorde's definitions of self-care. Overexercising, long commutes, toxic relationships, too much time spent indoors, and too much screen time are also common sources of stress. It will never be possible to completely avoid stressors, so when we can't decrease our exposure to them, we can instead focus on gaining mental and physical distance from their negative impacts.

You might be wondering, *How do self-care practices improve stress resilience?* Let's look at meditation, a self-care practice that can be done just about anywhere without needing to spend a dime. There are different kinds of meditation practices, but we'll focus on mindfulness meditation. Mindfulness is the act of being aware of the present moment— understanding what you're sensing, your thoughts, and your emotional state—without becoming overwhelmed and reactive. I like to think of mindfulness as a long stick that I can use to examine and turn over my emotions. I can approach an emotion—say, anger—with this long stick and look at it from different sides. I move the anger this way and that way and become curious about the sensation of anger. The shift from reactive to curious is the key.

Okay, so you're on your meditation cushion practicing attention and awareness, but what's happening in your brain? Research shows that practicing meditation activates brain regions involved in improved emotional control and modifies existing neural networks while also building new ones. If your brain is like a map with a road that ends in anger or anxiety (or other negative emotions), meditation revises that map, creating alternative roads so that you have multiple turns you can take away from anger and toward fewer negative thoughts or unhelpful reactions to stress.

One of the major differences between this kind of self-care and consumerism-based self-care is that mindfulness and meditation require practice and commitment. One way mindfulness specifically helps me navigate consumerism-based self-care is by encouraging me to pause and observe why I want something like, say, an expensive face serum. I tend to find out, when I pause and employ my curiosity, that I'm most likely tired and looking for a quick fix when what I need is rest. This isn't to say that I always resist the serum. After all, meditation is a lifelong practice for a reason: many other things vie for our attention. Ideally, a self-care practice promotes awareness of all those competing things and helps us navigate them without succumbing to overwhelming anxiety.

Food, movement, and self-care shape the bodies we inhabit, the world we live in, and how we live in it. Our lifestyle—or diet, as the ancient Greeks called it—matters more than any individual nutrient or specific exercise. All of the foods, movement practices, and ways we care for ourselves are what builds up the complex ecosystem of tissues and cells, muscles and bone, neurons and hormones that make us who we are.

A Brief History of Contraception & the Modern Options

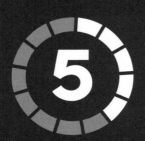

Ancient Greece provided us with a balanced and comprehensive definition of diet, but Hippocrates (460–375 BC) also recommended that if a woman didn't want to get pregnant after having sex, she should "jump so that the buttocks are touched by the feet." Vigorous jumping was meant to encourage the sperm to fall out of the vagina. Aristotle (384–322 BC) claimed that the embryo came from the seed of a man and the mother's only role in reproduction was nourishing that seed with her menstrual blood. Soranus (AD 98–138), the Greek physician, observed that conception was more likely if a woman had an orgasm. Thus, if she wished to avoid pregnancy, he said she should hold her breath when the man ejaculates, move away so the sperm can't penetrate her uterus, and "crouch down with bent knees and provoke sneezes."

Along with this very athletic and ineffective advice, the ancient Greeks did come up with a good option for avoiding both pregnancy and disease. Historians believe the first condom, made from the bladder of a goat, was used around 3000 BC by Pasiphaë, the wife of King Minos of Crete, whose semen was said to contain serpents and scorpions. Other cultures developed their own condoms: ancient Romans and Egyptians made them from linen and animals (sheep, goats, and calves); in China, the condom was made from silk paper; and the Japanese used tortoiseshells and leather.

It wasn't until 1858 that the first rubber condom emerged on the market. They were known as "American tips" because they only covered the glans of the penis. After a few decades of innovation, the modern condom—most often made of thin but strong latex that covers the whole penis—gained increasing popularity until the 1960s and 1970s when the birth control pill and copper and hormonal IUDs entered the market. Contraceptives were illegal until 1965, when they became legal for married couples. Seven years later, they became legal for unmarried people. The full controversial history, legality, stigma, and availability of various types of contraceptives can and does fill many books (see resources on page 254). For now, let's look at how contraceptive development overlapped with the science of fertility—including how conception works and when it's possible for a pregnancy to occur.

In 1678, the "father of microbiology," Antonie van Leeuwenhoek, used a microscope to observe his own semen and discovered tiny swimming sperm in his personal sample. In 1868, the observation of cervical secretions revealed that the translucent, clear secretions with the consistency of raw egg white encouraged sperm migration. In 1869, scientists uncovered that body temperature fluctuates throughout the menstrual cycle. Mary Putnam Jacobi, the physician who challenged the sexist Edward H. Clarke, furthered the research on basal body temperature fluctuations. She discovered that body temperature went up many days before menstruation, but didn't link the change in temperature to ovulation.

While van Leeuwenhoek and other men observed their sperm swimming merrily under microscopes for a few hundred years, it wasn't until 1928 that Edgar Allen, the same guy who collected pregnant women's urine and first isolated estrogen, discovered that within ovarian follicles is the egg. In the same year, the mythology of the twenty-eight-day cycle was questioned by the Swiss gynecologist Rudolf Vollman. He believed that people with "regular" menstrual cycles only existed in medical textbooks and that other biophysical measurements more accurately predicted ovulation.

Before the expansion of contraceptive options in the 1960s, condoms and fertility awareness-based methods like the calendar and rhythm method were popular. Then in 1995, Allen Wilcox used hormonal assays to show that conception can happen during a six-day window, and new methods involving measuring, observing, and tracking biomarkers of fertile days of the menstrual cycle became part of fertility awareness-based methods.

We now have an increased understanding of the science of reproduction along with many options for managing our reproductive health. However, this science and these options aren't equally available to all people. In her article "No, Drinking Hot Water or Jumping Vigorously After Sex Won't Prevent Pregnancy," the health care educator Jane Otai wrote that young girls ages eleven to fifteen in Nairobi explained to her that they knew how to avoid getting pregnant and their strategies didn't include contraception or abstinence. Instead, they recommended, "taking a hot bath, drinking hot water, jumping vigorously after sex, having sex in a standing position, or having sex when it is raining or in a swimming pool."

This misunderstanding of reproductive biology isn't a Nairobi-specific problem. When people aren't taught about reproductive health, the risk for sexually transmitted diseases, unintended pregnancy, and poor pregnancy outcomes increases. Better education is one piece of the puzzle, but the other essential piece is our socioecological context, which connects how individual, interpersonal, community, and social structures determine health at the level of the population. Systemic and institutionalized racism places racially oppressed groups, specifically Black women, at much higher risk for negative health outcomes such as maternal death. Racism and population-based oppression is an issue of reproductive and feminist justice, and sexual and reproductive health equity and freedom are human rights that everyone must fight for at each level of our socioecological system.

The next sections focus on contraceptive options including hormonal birth control methods, barrier methods like condoms, and fertility awareness-based methods. The best contraception is the one that effectively prevents pregnancy and fits into your lifestyle and preferences. And while we'll look in-depth at fertility awareness-based methods, this book is not pushing any one form of contraception over any others. What matters is that what you choose works and it works for you.

The Ins and Outs of Reproduction

First, let's cover some basic reproductive information including how long sperm survive in the genital tract, the timing of ovulation, and how long after ovulation fertilization can still occur. The lifespan of sperm is seven days; however, most sperm live about three days on average. Eggs can live for twenty-four hours and the average lifespan of an egg is seventeen hours. For a sperm and egg to unite and become an eventual embryo, the lifespan of the egg and sperm must overlap. The most likely days of conception are within a six-day fertile window, with peak conception rates the day before ovulation and the day of ovulation.

The timing of ovulation is variable between individuals, variable from cycle to cycle in the same individuals, and influenced by multiple factors, so it isn't useful or accurate to rely on an average twenty-eight-day calendar method to predict your unique fertile window. The effectiveness of various methods of contraception is measured using estimated failure rates based on perfect use and typical use. Perfect use means the contraception is employed exactly as intended. For example, taking the birth control pill every day at the same time and never missing a day. Typical use is how most use contraceptives (other than the ones that are implanted) and accounts for mistakes, inconsistency, or misuse. For example, missing a pill or using a condom inconsistently or applied ineffectively are examples of typical use. For context, abstinence is the *only* method of contraception with a 0 percent failure rate while contraceptives such as IUDs, hormone implants, and injections have a failure rate under 1 percent while the birth control pill has a 7 percent failure rate with typical use and condoms have a typical use failure rate of 13 percent. Depending on the type of method used and the user, the typical use failure rate range for fertility awareness-based methods is 2–23 percent according to the CDC.

Conception Probability

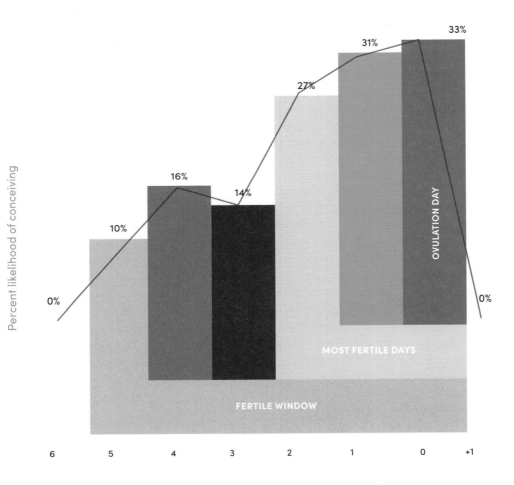

Percent likelihood of conceiving

0%

10%

16%

14%

27%

31%

33%

0%

OVULATION DAY

MOST FERTILE DAYS

FERTILE WINDOW

6   5   4   3   2   1   0   +1

Day of intercourse relative to ovulation

The Hormones

At the time of this writing, the types of hormonal birth control methods on the market include the pill, patches, shots, implants, and hormonal IUDs. The birth control pill is the most popular and widely used form of contraception in the United States. The three major categories are the combined pill, which contains estrogen and progestin; progestin-only pills, also known as POPs or minipills; and extended use pills, which contain estrogen and progestin, but are used continuously, greatly reducing or eliminating the number of periods per year.

Hormonal birth control is safe for most people who menstruate, and it's effective at preventing pregnancy. Like any medicine, it carries risks and benefits. Side effects include breakthrough bleeding, breast tenderness, nausea, mood changes, and headaches. Combined oral contraceptives increase the risk of deep vein thrombosis, stroke, and heart attack in some people. The benefits include effective contraception, obviously, and hormonal birth control is also used for noncontraceptive benefits such as the treatment of acne, endometriosis-related pain, PCOS, menstrual-related migraines, PMS, and ovarian cysts and fibroids. Finally, according to research, the use of combined oral contraceptives lowers the risk of colorectal, endometrial, and ovarian cancer while *slightly* increasing the risk of breast and cervical cancer.

Hormonal contraceptives prevent ovulation and/or thicken cervical mucus, which stops sperm from passing through the cervix. In a sense, they trick your body into believing it's pregnant. During the luteal phase and throughout pregnancy, high levels of natural progesterone and estrogen travel in the bloodstream to receptors in the pituitary and stop it from releasing the hormones that orchestrate ovulation. Hormonal contraceptives provide a continuous dose of synthetic (exogenous) progestins and estrogen, which stops the pituitary from telling the ovaries to produce the natural (endogenous) ebb and flow of estrogen and progesterone.

With most formulations of hormonal contraceptives, especially combination birth control pills, ovulation is suppressed, and the "period" is technically a bleed that happens in response to a withdrawal from the hormones in the pill. This is different from menstrual bleeding when a person is off hormonal contraceptives because the pill prevents the endometrial lining from thickening, so the bleeding is often lighter, and it's possible to experience only spotting or no bleeding on the days the person takes inactive pills. Because the pill suppresses ovulation, the physical biomarkers of ovulation, like fertile cervical mucus, are generally

Hormone Comparison

HORMONE CHANGES IN AN AVERAGE CYCLE

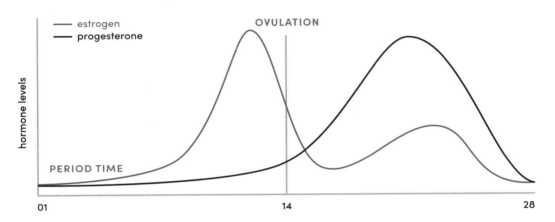

— estrogen
— progesterone

OVULATION

PERIOD TIME

hormone levels

01   14   28

HORMONE LEVELS FOR PEOPLE USING
COMBINATION HORMONAL CONTRACEPTIVES

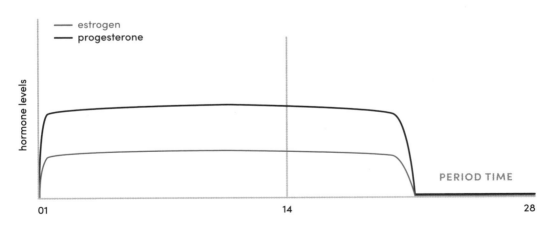

— estrogen
— progesterone

hormone levels

PERIOD TIME

01   14   28

not observable, but it is worthwhile to track side effects such as mood and breakthrough bleeding when using this method. There are so many choices available that if you prefer to use hormonal contraceptives, but don't like the one you're currently using, you are very likely to find one that works better for you.

The Barriers

Condoms, diaphragms, cervical caps, and sponges act as barriers between sperm and egg. Male and female condoms are the only forms of birth control methods that protect against sexually transmitted infections (STIs). They are less effective at preventing pregnancy than hormonal contraceptives; in health class, they teach us to put condoms on bananas for a reason: they don't work well if you don't use them the right way. For people using hormonal contraceptives or practicing fertility awareness-based methods, condoms play an essential role in STI prevention and pregnancy prevention during the fertile window.

Copper IUDs, like levonorgestrel (a synthetic progestin)-containing IUDs but without added hormones, are long-term, reversible, intrauterine devices that are extremely effective at preventing pregnancy. These small, copper-coated T-shaped devices prevent sperm from joining with an egg and make it harder for a fertilized egg to implant in the uterus.

The Emergency Meds

There are three options available for emergency contraception to prevent possible pregnancy. First, a person could get a copper IUD, which is the most effective form of emergency contraception (EC). If placed within 120 hours, or five days, of having unprotected sex, it is 99.9 percent effective at preventing pregnancy. Second, a person could take EC pills including ulipristal acetate (brand name ella and the most effective EC pill with up to five days of efficacy) and levonorgestrel (brand name Plan B One-Step and known as "the morning after pill"), which is effective up to three days. Thirdly, if these options aren't available, some combination birth control pills can be used in higher dosages, known as the Yuzpe method (talk to your doctor for guidance). These options work best the sooner they are taken after unprotected intercourse with a sperm-contributing partner. Importantly, EC pills are not abortion medications. They work by preventing ovulation, and if an embryo is already implanted, EC pills will not harm an existing pregnancy. Note that EC pills are less effective for those who weigh over 155 pounds and may not work at all for people over 195 pounds. IUDs, on the other hand, are effective for people at any weight.

The Tracking

Fertility awareness–based methods (FAM) either use a single indicator or a combination of indicators including temperature, cervical mucus, cervical position, and cycle length to identify the fertile window. FAM is often used to become pregnant or to prevent pregnancy by predicting ovulation and avoiding, or pursuing, sex with a sperm-contributing partner the five days leading up to ovulation (the lifespan of sperm) and the day of ovulation (the lifespan of the egg). Combined symptothermal methods (tracking both temperature and signs of ovulation like cervical mucus and position) have the highest rate of effectiveness at pregnancy prevention, but they also require daily measurement and charting, which can be burdensome and isn't for everyone.

FAM is commonly referred to as "family planning," but observing and tracking the menstrual cycle is not only for people in relationships and it doesn't need to be used as a form of contraception; it can also be used to pay attention to your body while you use other methods of contraception. For people with irregular cycles, those with multiple sexual partners, or people who *really* don't want to become pregnant, a second method of contraception, such as the tried-and-true condom, is essential. If you are interested in using FAM as contraception or just curious about the physical signs of ovulation, see the next three sections on cervical mucus, basal body temperature, and cervical positioning.

Magical Mucus

The main reproductive targets for estrogen and progesterone include the endometrium, cervix, and breasts. During the follicular phase when the hypothalamus tells the pituitary to release FSH and LH and these hormones call down to the follicles to secrete estrogen and release an egg, the initial rise in estrogen followed by progesterone influences the type of mucus secreted by the cells lining the cervix. Sperm motility is either encouraged or impeded by the quality, quantity, and composition of cervical secretions. During the early follicular phase and luteal phase, the cervix produces either scant, minimal secretions or thick, sticky, white secretions. In this highly acidic environment, sperm are quickly destroyed and not allowed to enter the reproductive tract.

As estrogen levels climb and ovulation approaches, the secretions transform. The increased water content and altered mucin structure result in secretions that gradually become more transparent, wetter, stretchier, and more passable for sperm. The wettest, most transparent, slipperiest, and stickiest day, when your secretions are described as having the consistency of egg white and you can stretch them apart with your fingers, is known as peak day and closely coincides with ovulation. You know you experienced peak day when the following day, your secretions once again become white, thick, and sticky, which is antagonizing to sperm and marks the end of the fertile window.

For most people, it takes around three cycles of observing and tracking cervical secretions before they feel confident identifying the changes through the cycle and peak day. This means caution and attention are paramount whenever we start observing our signs of fertility. Observing cervical secretions includes feeling and looking. First, feeling. Note whether you feel generally wet or dry. Do your external vaginal secretions feel sticky or slippery or thick and lotiony? You may also feel more easily and naturally aroused and interested in sex when your cervical secretions become more slippery. Next, looking. Are your secretions white or clear? Notice the discharge on your underwear or after going to the bathroom and wiping. What does the fluid look like? Keep track of your mucus throughout the day, paying attention to how you feel and what the fluid looks like each time you go to the bathroom or when you change your clothes. This daily observation gives you the information to record when you track your cervical secretions. Here is a timeline of cervical mucus as it corresponds to the phases of the menstrual cycle.

1. **MENSTRUAL PHASE:** This is the bleeding phase, and as your endometrium sheds, the cervix produces few secretions. During this phase, track and record your bleeding patterns.

2. **FOLLICULAR/PREOVULATORY PHASE:**

   EARLY FOLLICULAR: Following the bleeding phase, estrogen slowly starts to rise but low levels lead to minimal or absent secretions. Note whether your secretions are absent or minimal and if you feel dry.

LATE FOLLICULAR: As estrogen levels climb, the quantity of secretions increases and tends to look and feel sticky, white, and creamy. This is when you might note a thicker, lotion-like consistency of mucus.

3. **OVULATORY PHASE:** As ovulation approaches, increasing amounts of secretions take on a translucent, stretchy, and slippery look and feel. One to two days before you ovulate, as estrogen levels surge, cervical secretions may take on the classic egg-white appearance and consistency and your vagina feels wetter. Not everyone experiences this egg-white mucus. When water content is higher, your mucus may just feel slippery and wet and look clear but not stretch between your fingers. This is still fertile mucus! This cervical mucus encourages sperm motility into the reproductive tract and creates an alkaline environment to promote sperm survival.

4. **LUTEAL PHASE:** One to two days after ovulation, when progesterone enters the scene, cervical secretions are inhibited and become sticky, dry, or minimal until menstruation occurs again.

Cervical secretions are not the only fluids that come out of the vagina. Arousal fluid is wet, clear, and slippery. Sexual arousal increases the blood flow to the genitals, which triggers certain glands and the cervix to release fluid that lubricates the vagina. Generally, during the reproductive years, increased arousal leads to more vaginal lubrication, which dissipates within about an hour of intercourse. Tracking your cycle should always include when you had sex and if it was with a sperm-contributing partner, whether or not you used additional contraception.

Certain medical conditions and infections can change or interfere with cervical secretions. PCOS (polycystic ovarian syndrome), recent pregnancies and breastfeeding, dehydration, reproductive tract infections, IUDs, hormonal birth control, and other medications are a few examples that alter vaginal discharge and cervical mucus quality, quantity, and composition. Abnormal vaginal discharge represents a disruption in the vaginal ecosystem and should also be tracked. Grayish, thick, chunky/cheesy, yellowish, green, fishy, or off-smelling discharge indicates a disruption in normal healthy secretions and may be caused by yeast infections, bacterial infections, and/or sexually transmitted infections. Genital pain, itching, burning, soreness, swelling, and redness often accompany these symptoms. If you are experiencing these signs and symptoms, visit your health care provider. Because cervical mucus is the most important biomarker of fertility and also because it can sometimes be

Cervical Mucus and Ovulation

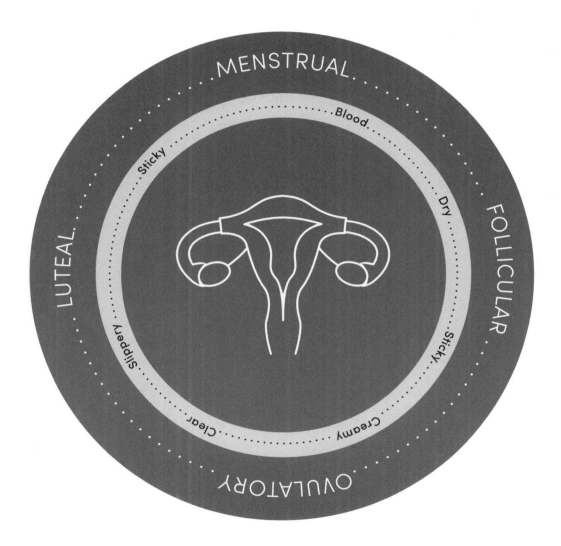

tricky to learn to track, you may benefit greatly from working with a fertility awareness educator, especially during transitions in your life like during the return of fertility after pregnancy.

Thermoregulated and Proud

Early studies on thermoregulation, the way the body maintains core body temperature, focused entirely on cisgender men. Women were excluded from this research because of a general assumption that they were less physically active, and thus less fit, compared to men. Scientists also assumed that women didn't have the physiological capacity to acclimate to fluctuations in external temperature. These assumptions turned out to be false. Humans of all genders are remarkably capable of maintaining core body temperature within a few tenths of a degree. However, the physiology and biology of people who ovulate are one step more intricate and interesting. People who don't ovulate experience monophasic, or consistent core body temperatures, while people who do ovulate experience biphasic core body temperatures with lower body temperature before ovulation and higher core body temperature after ovulation.

Both at rest and during exercise, progesterone and estrogen influence thermoregulation and body temperature. One of the main functions of our ovarian hormones is to create an environment in the body that is friendly to conception and fetal growth; a temperature-controlled environment is part of what makes a uterus appealing to a potential embryo. When it comes to tracking basal body temperature (BBT), what we're specifically paying attention to is the patterns of our preovulatory and postovulatory core body temperatures. After ovulation, when progesterone rises, we experience what is called a sustained thermal shift.

The thermal shift is subtle, increasing BBT by about 0.5°F to 1.0°F (0.3°C to 0.6°C). This measurement can come from the vagina, armpit, or mouth and requires a sensitive thermometer, specifically a digital or basal body thermometer that goes to two decimal places, or tenth-degree accuracy. These thermometers range in form and price from simple thermometers to wearable technology. Because talking, moving, and eating increase body temperature, BBT must be taken every day, at the same time, immediately in the morning before you get out of bed and after at least five hours of sleep. In her book *The Fifth Vital Sign*, the fertility awareness expert Lisa Hendrickson-Jack recommends leaving the thermometer in place for ten minutes before taking your temperature. This extra step helps her clients get more consistent, stable, and accurate temperature readings with fewer dips and spikes in their charts since the thermometer has time to stabilize and warm up.

Unlike cervical mucus, which can tell you whether you're fertile or not in the moment, BBT is useful for retrospectively tracking ovulation and gauging overall health and fertility. For this reason, many Traditional Chinese Medicine doctors who focus on fertility evaluate BBT charts with every menstrual cycle to confirm ovulation and evaluate overall health. External factors such as stress, environmental toxins, going to bed too late, restless sleep, a poor diet, and drinking alcohol can cause temperature spikes or irregularities that negatively affect egg development and the timing of ovulation.

The other interrupters of BBT include certain medications, illnesses, and diseases; traveling and jet lag; and other disruptors of our sleep like shift work, screens, bright lights, and low exposure to natural light. Our body temperature fluctuates with our circadian rhythm and with an ovulatory menstrual cycle. These two cycles are related. The hormones that govern our sleep and those that mediate reproductive function influence basic body functions like thermoregulation and metabolism. The relationship between the menstrual cycle and circadian rhythm is bidirectional and interactive. This means that our circadian rhythm is altered by the menstrual cycle and a disrupted circadian rhythm is associated with menstrual cycle irregularities and disturbances.

Tracking BBT every day might seem like a hassle. But part of charting is understanding that life happens, and our charts should have room for notes and details that provide us with essential information about our lifestyle and patterns. BBT, when tracked consistently, can provide us with clues to our health. We might see greater temperature variations or changes in our cycle length when we're going through a particularly stressful period in our life or when our sleep is disrupted. These clues give us the tools to understand how our lifestyle impacts our basic metabolic and reproductive health, and crucially, they allow us to experiment on ourselves with improved diet, sleep hygiene, movement, and stress management and notice changes. This information is empowerment in our hands, data that applies to us alone and that we have the capacity to influence through our choices. The persistent myth of our culture is that the health of people who have menstrual cycles is too messy and unimportant to study. But, by simply checking your temperature once a day, you can offer a subtle yet profound f-you to the science that historically neglected our physiology.

Here are a few essential points for BBT tracking and charting:

1. Use a BBT thermometer and choose whether you want to take your temperature vaginally, orally, or under your armpit. Stick to this location.

2. In an ideal world, measure BBT after at least five hours of sleep before getting out of bed in the morning at the same time each day. If your process gets disrupted, note the time of day and variance next to your temperature.

3. Hold the thermometer in place for ten minutes before taking your temperature.

4. Three consecutive temperatures in a row that are higher than the previous six indicate ovulation occurred.

5. The typical normal range for preovulatory BBT is 97 to 97.5°F (36.11 to 36.36°C) and postovulatory BBT is usually 97.6°F to 98.6°F (36.44 to 37°C).

6. Understand that there is no perfect BBT chart and disruptions are a normal part of life. Continue to track and chart through the cycles and phases of life.

7. A sustained high BBT for eighteen days after ovulation may indicate pregnancy.

8. Use cervical mucus (see page 50) and cervical positioning (below) in addition to BBT. The combined indicator approach is more accurate and effective.

Meet Your Cervix

Connecting the body of the uterus to the vagina, the cervix is around three to four centimeters long and mostly composed of connective tissue and muscle. The cervix serves several purposes. It protects the uterus from viruses and bacteria and secretes the mucus you can monitor. The mix of muscle and connective tissues allows the cervix to close tightly or dilate either a little or a lot to allow cervical mucus, sperm, menstrual blood, or a baby to pass through.

Throughout the cycle, the feeling and position of the cervix change. For most of the menstrual cycle, the cervix is a firm and closed structure that feels like the tip of your nose. Its position is fairly low in the vagina, but as you approach ovulation, the cervix softens, opens, and moves deeper, or higher, into the vagina. Instead of a nose, the cervix may now feel more like pursed lips or an earlobe. The cervix, just like the rest of the reproductive system, responds to increasing levels of estrogen by maneuvering into a position that is more receptive for sex and conception. Noticing cervical position and feeling changes in its texture requires consistent, hands-on palpation. Feeling your cervix every day is the best way to become familiar with the unique and subtle ways your cervix changes throughout the menstrual cycle.

Like basal body temperature, cervical position gives us retrospective information about when we ovulated and is best used in combination with cervical mucus and BBT tracking. Follow these steps to learn how to feel your cervix and track the changes.

1. Thoroughly wash your hands and get into a squatting position or place one foot higher up on a stool or the side of the bathtub if you're in the shower.

2. Insert your middle finger into your vagina. Gently move your finger deeper until you feel the cervix toward the back of your vagina where the walls are soft and supple. If you move your finger in a circle, you should be able to feel your cervix and the middle opening, the os.

3. Note how your cervix feels. Soft or firm, wet or dry? Does it feel squishy and receptive or closed? Does your cervix feel high or low?

4. Remember, experience and practice will allow you to comfortably assess your cervix. Practice daily and write down what you feel.

See the resources on page 254 for recommended fertility awareness-based tracking methods including apps, journals, and books.

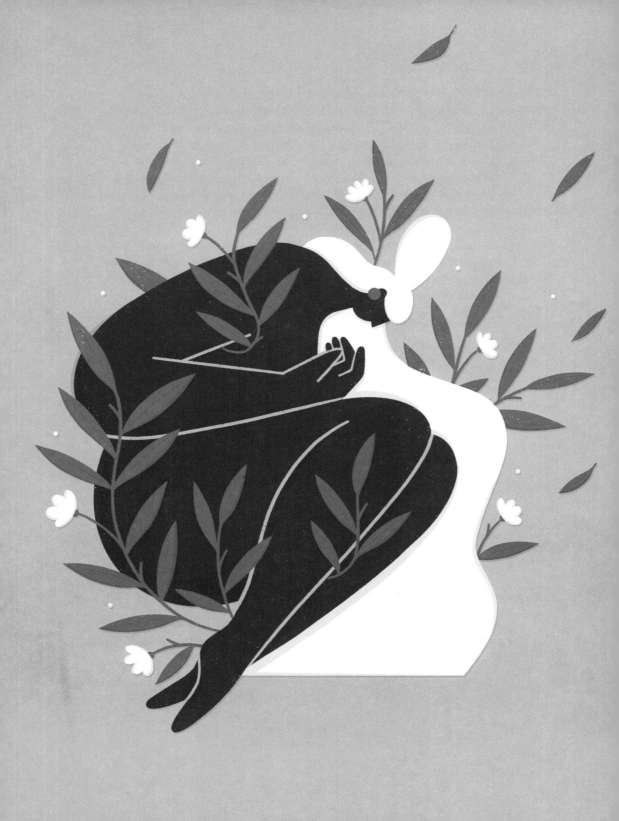

PART TWO

The Four Seasons of Your Cycle

Throughout history, diverse cultures have linked life cycles and processes to seasons, viewing them as metaphors for change and exemplars of the connection between our inner ecology and the world around us. The phases of the menstrual cycle are often understood as their own seasons because seasons are tangible moments in time that represent transition and they are also rich in symbolism. This symbolism gives seasons a sense of meaning and feeling that line up extraordinarily well with how we experience our cycles.

By viewing each phase of the menstrual cycle as its own season and correlating this season with those we experience in nature, you might notice that you feel more connected and gentler with yourself. For example, if you feel like curling up at home in sweatpants, eating warm food, and resting during the menstrual phase, thinking of this phase as winter for the body helps you understand why you might desire extra coziness. Integrating seasonal metaphors into the way we understand the menstrual cycle also gives us language to describe the fluctuations happening internally. We can't see how we feel or what's happening in the uterus, but we can imagine and see leaves dropping from a tree in the fall or a garden growing in the springtime. This visual, metaphorical language has the potential to deeply connect us to our own physical sensations and the natural world that surrounds us through the power of awareness and observation.

In the next four chapters, we'll explore the biological and sociocultural aspects as well as the subtler, more symbolic properties of each phase of the menstrual cycle. Each chapter is accompanied by ten approachable recipes that support your physiological needs during that phase of your cycle. Additionally, each chapter contains guidance for movement and self-care rituals to nourish your mind and body. This section is the nuts and bolts of the book, containing information that you can return to over and over again as you cycle through each season.

Cycle Seasons

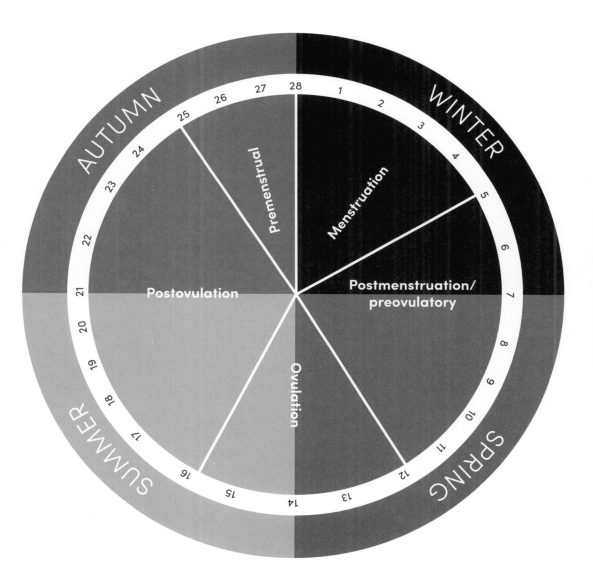

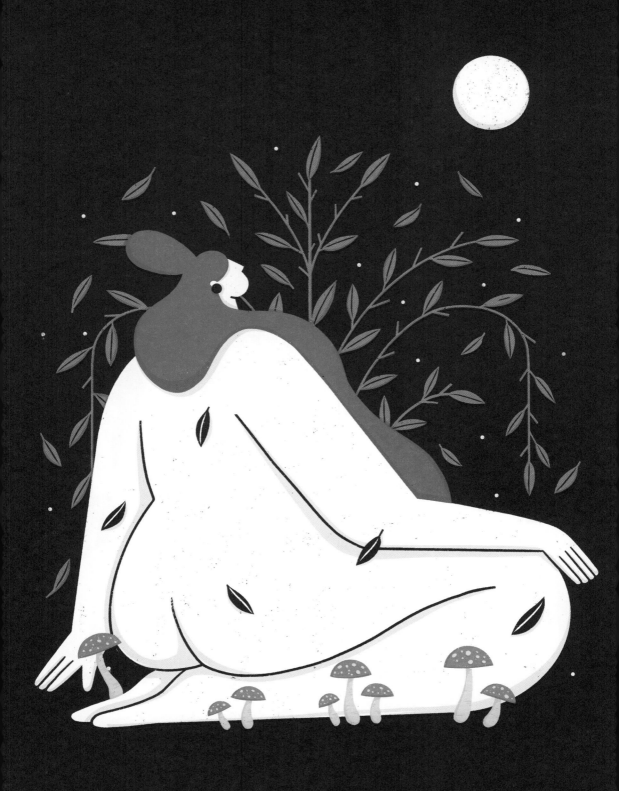

Menstrual Phase

WINTER • REST + REFLECT

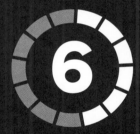

To survive snowfall and cold temperatures during the winter, deciduous trees enter a state of dormancy similar to hibernation. Beginning in late fall, the leaves detach, and the tree's growth and metabolism slow down. Through incredible adaptations and coping mechanisms—like changing cell membrane pliability to withstand freezing temperatures—trees not only survive winter, but they also plan for winter by sensing changes in the weather and conserving sugars and other nutrients for the cold months ahead. The trees don't die when they shed their leaves or during winter. They slow down; they take a break. Under their blanket of snow, trees quietly offer us humans many lessons about how to prepare for and adapt to winter, both the season and as a metaphor for our internal process of shedding and regeneration.

The cycle of loss, adaptation, and ultimately, survival is a rhythm that plants, animals, and humans live by. Ancient cultures devised rituals during winter that were centered on opposites like darkness and light, yin and yang, stagnation and regeneration. These rituals were, ultimately, about life and hope during the challenges brought on by winter. The menstrual cycle is often described as a season of inner winter for the body or a type of death cycle, as winter is characterized not only by death but also by rebirth. In chapter one, we explored why we bleed in the context of evolutionary biology. One of the leading theories discussed there is that we have choosy uteri that cyclically shed and regenerate the inner portion of the endometrium to give us every advantage at reproductive success and personal survival. This process of inflammation and tissue breakdown of the inner layer of the uterus, which then subsequently repairs and regenerates, is nothing short of remarkable. It allows our bodies to let go of the past and prepare for the future.

Despite the reality that menstruation is a remarkable process of loss followed by rapid renewal, people like Edward H. Clarke, Aristotle, and many others viewed menstruation as a sign of inferiority. This opinion weakens as more voices speak out and speak louder against the stigma and oppression associated with menstruation. In the 1960s, when some men were opposed to women holding positions of power in part because of their menstrual cycles, the renowned endocrinologist Estelle Ramage countered that instead of being a symbol of inferiority, menstruation is proof of female strength. She said, "In man, the shedding of blood is always associated with injury, disease, or death. Only the female half of humanity is seen to have the magical ability to bleed profusely and still rise phoenix-like each month from the gore."

Menstruation is a process of simultaneous demolition and remodeling of the uterus. The demolition starts with a steep progesterone withdrawal. This withdrawal tells other workers like inflammatory mediators and leukocytes to get to work on breaking down and shedding the luminal layer of the uterus. Even as shedding occurs, repairs begin. Cells start building a new luminal surface on menstrual day two and completely cover the lumen by day six. Progesterone is thought to initiate both the process of demolition and repair, overseeing the project of the uterus makeover like an architect with utter faith in their vision.

Just as important as the biology of menstruation is the language we use to describe it because language shapes our experience. The way we talk, or don't talk, about menstruation matters. The linguist Dr. Elizabeth Kissling writes, "Experience is always mediated through language and interaction. Our own embodiment, seemingly the most 'real' and concrete experience humans have, cannot be known directly but only by speaking and thinking about it." The messages we receive about menstruation set us up to feel a sense of internal conflict about our cycles. The result is a feeling of alienation from our bodies and an understanding that menstruation is something to dread. Of this problem of language and the menstrual cycle, Kissling writes, "menstruation is represented in education materials and parental talk as part of women's unique and valuable physiological capacity for childbearing, but portrayed in advertisements and in some women's and girls' conversations as 'the curse,' one of the least pleasurable aspects of being female."

The menstrual cycle isn't a curse or a punishment; it is a reproductive function. And our experience, good or bad, gives us meaningful insight into our overall health. Our cultural narrative explains the menstrual cycle as something that just happens to us and encourages distance from the experience. But paying attention to and acknowledging how we feel throughout our cycle encourage a sense of closeness and ownership of our reproductive health. Perhaps the best challenge for this experiment on changing our minds is our blood. Unlike other parts of our physiology that we learn about, but can't see, menstruating isn't abstract. Nothing reminds us of the realness of this experience quite like the blood. In this next section, we'll examine the details of the flow.

Blood and Cycle Basics

The bleeding phase lasts for three to seven days, and we bleed, on average, 35 to 50 mL (7 to 10 teaspoons); however, blood loss can vary from 5 mL to 80 mL. The normal range of bleeding includes 5 mL, but this is an extremely low amount of blood and may suggest low hormone levels, a thin endometrial lining, or other issues with the menstrual cycle. On the other hand, bleeding more than 80 mL or for longer than seven days is described as *menorrhagia*, or heavy periods, and is associated with menstrual cycle irregularities such as endometriosis, uterine fibroids, or endocrine dysfunction. Spotting may occur a day or two before or after your period, but continuous bleeding throughout the rest of your cycle is not normal and requires medical evaluation. Besides using a menstrual cup to measure how much you're bleeding, you can also approximate how much you're bleeding by keeping track of how often you need to change your pad, tampon, or period underwear. You are experiencing a heavy menstrual period if your flow soaks through your tampon or pad every hour for multiple hours, if you need to change your pad or tampon at night, and if you pass multiple grape (or larger) size clots.

The color of menstrual blood depends on how long that blood has been exposed to oxygen and changes over the course of your period. Prior to menstruating, spiral arteries, which supply blood to the part of the endometrium that sheds, constrict and cause the endometrium to become ischemic. This lack of oxygen supply triggers the sloughing of the endometrium, but not all at once. Early blood may leave the body slowly and appear brownish, dark red, black, or bright red. Bright red blood tends to characterize the heavier bleeding on the second and third days of your period as the uterine lining sheds more quickly. As your period progresses, the hue may shift to dark red, especially near the end of bleeding. Then, as your bleeding tapers off, you may see brownish or black blood reappear. Blood clots tend to show up on the heaviest days of menstruation and may appear dark red or black. Like color, the consistency and texture of blood may change throughout your period. Bright red blood tends to be viscous, not too thin, and not too thick, while the early or late brown blood may be more spotty, thin, or streaky.

You might be surprised to learn that it isn't just blood. It is a complex biological fluid composed of blood, endometrial cells, vaginal secretions, enzymes, proteins from immune cells, and microbes. Menstrual blood has another ingredient that medicine is excited about: mesenchymal-like stem cells. Stem cells are able to self-renew and differentiate into various specialized cell types. Most stem cells studied in medical research come from bone marrow (the gold standard), umbilical cord blood, endometrial tissue, adipose tissue, dental pulp, and other sites that require invasive methods like surgery to obtain. Accessing menstrual blood mesenchymal-like stem cells is noninvasive and several preclinical studies show that they are effective in preventing and controlling various issues such as diabetes, liver disease, wounds, and tissue damage.

Clinical guidelines tell us that the average menstrual cycle length is twenty-eight days, almost always in the twenty-five to thirty-day range, with ovulation occurring around day fourteen and a fourteen-day-long luteal phase. Until recently, there hasn't been much data to dispute this accepted definition of a "normal" menstrual cycle. However, as more people use apps that record cycle details, more data is available than ever before, and what all that data tells us is that from person to person, menstrual cycles are defined more by their variability than their adherence to averages. The timing of ovulation, bleeding duration, and the length of the follicular phase varies among individuals and changes as we age. For example, in a 2019 study from *Nature*, data from more than six hundred thousand menstrual cycles showed that age is negatively correlated with cycle length, meaning that as we get older, our cycles tend to get shorter. The average cycle length for all ages was 29.3 days plus or minus 5.2 days. From age twenty-five to forty-five, cycle length dropped by 3.2 days, follicular phase length dropped by 3.4 days, and bleeding duration also decreased. The biggest variation the study found was in the duration of the follicular phase, which is generally assumed to be fourteen days. Instead, the study showed the average follicular phase was 16.9 days. Individuals with longer cycles (31–35 days) averaged a follicular phase of 19.5 days while those with shorter cycles (21–24 days) averaged a follicular phase of 12.4 days.

The huge range of normal cycles highlights the inherent variability between individuals and how important it is to track your unique biomarkers of fertility. And while there is variation in normal cycles, irregular menstrual cycles—cycles that are not within five to seven days cycle to cycle, or very long menstrual cycles—are associated with an increased risk of premature mortality before age seventy due to conditions like cancer and cardiovascular disease. This finding came from a 2020 study published in the *British Medical Journal* that compared cisgender women with irregular or long menstrual cycles with those who had regular or short cycles. The menstrual cycle reflects the functioning of the hypothalamic-pituitary-ovarian (HPO) axis. Individuals with irregular or long cycles are likely experiencing a disrupted hormonal environment, and they are more likely to have insulin resistance, which inhibits sex hormone binding globulin (SHBG) and leads to higher levels of free testosterone and estrogen. This may then contribute to the development of cancer, diabetes, cardiovascular disease, and PCOS. This study provides more evidence that it's worth paying attention to the signs our cycles give us about our internal hormonal environment. During our reproductive years, our menstrual cycle—its length and regularity—acts as a proxy for our overall health.

A BRIEF HISTORY OF FEMCARE

While we're talking about bleeding, let's take a look at menstrual care products. Historically these products have been labeled "feminine hygiene" products or "femcare." While menstrual care products are obviously useful and necessary, the history of femcare marketing has benefited from telling people who menstruate that disposable and "hygiene" products are the key to freedom while meticulously maintaining period stigmas and taboos. The first disposable menstrual care products emerged in 1921; pads came first, then tampons. Tampons were initially a tricky sell because doctors and parents were disturbed by the idea of young women touching their genitals. The applicator was designed as a tool to uphold young girls' innocence lest they be tempted to look or touch *down there* when they put in a tampon. Cardboard, glass, and stainless steel were used as applicators before flexible plastic stole the show as the applicator material of choice. Soon after, plastic found its way into the absorbent material, the strings on the ends of tampons, and the packages enclosing individual tampons. Quiet plastic wrappers were developed to "help keep it a secret." Millions of plastic applicators end up in the ocean ecosystem and on beaches where kids find them and think they are whistles. Companies selling these unsustainable products continue to benefit from our ingrained desire to hide our periods, even if that means the products of our discretion persist in our environment for five hundred years after a single use.

Along with plastic came synthetic chemicals. A study in 2019 found that many different brands of menstrual products come laden with chemicals such as volatile organic compounds (VOCs) and phthalates. These toxic chemicals are linked to endocrine disruption, cancer, reproductive health problems, and nervous system damage. Since these products are in contact with the external genitalia for long periods of time, they are more likely to be absorbed into the reproductive system. In 2020, New York became the first state to require ingredient disclosure on menstrual product packaging with the passing of the Menstrual Products Right to Know Act. Other states have started to introduce bills regarding menstrual product access and ingredient disclosure.

The year 2020 seems a little late to have a right to know what's in the products we use, but it's a good sign of the cultural shift happening in our attitudes toward our periods. The options for non-toxic, reusable, biodegradable, and sustainable menstrual care products are expanding. Before the use of branded disposables, scraps of reusable fabric and other absorbent materials were commonplace, and a menstrual cup was first introduced in the 1930s. Improved versions of older products like reusable pads, period-proof underwear, and menstrual cups represent a wave of innovation that has been lacking in the menstrual care industry for the last century.

Addressing Painful Periods

Dysmenorrhea, or painful periods, is incredibly common and the leading cause of absence from work and school among people who menstruate during their reproductive years. Additionally, people with painful periods, compared to those without painful periods, report enhanced pain sensitivity and are at a higher risk of developing other chronic pain conditions. There is great individual variability in how we experience dysmenorrhea, but symptoms include abdominal cramping; pain in the lower back, legs, head, and vagina; gastrointestinal symptoms like vomiting, gas, and diarrhea; or severe body-wide pain. Dysmenorrhea is most likely caused by hormone-like compounds called prostaglandins that increase immediately before menstruation and increase vasoconstriction and cramping in uterine tissue. Studies have found that people with dysmenorrhea have higher levels of prostaglandins than those without period-related pain and this causes increased inflammation and stronger, more painful menstrual cramping. Along with prostaglandins, some studies show that people with dysmenorrhea have disrupted uterine blood flow and that menstruation exacerbates underlying health issues. The authors of one study concluded that dysmenorrhea is not just a disorder of the menstrual phase but also an indicator of a disorder of the whole menstrual cycle.

The most common treatments for period-related pain are nonsteroidal anti-inflammatory drugs (NSAIDs) like ibuprofen and oral contraceptive pills. NSAIDs are backed by the most robust research supporting their ability to reduce dysmenorrhea. They do so by inhibiting prostaglandin synthesis, which lessens the severity of menstrual cramps. When menstrual cramps are debilitating, NSAIDs can quickly relieve the pain and reduce the heaviness of the menstrual flow (when used consistently).

Treatments for dysmenorrhea vary based on symptoms and personal preferences, and on pages 71–72, you'll find holistic, non-pharmacological recommendations for relief that are both anecdotally supported and evidence-based for treating period pain. For some people, NSAIDs or hormonal contraceptives effectively relieve their pain, while others may find that exercise, eating more protein, fruits, and vegetables, eating smaller portion sizes, and hydrating help alleviate symptoms. Movement is particularly effective at reducing pain because it increases blood flow and metabolism of the uterus, which can decrease menstrual pain and release endorphins. Endorphins are secreted by the brain and change our perception of pain by increasing our pain threshold. Certain types of movements, which you'll see on page 78, help reduce tension in the ligamentous bands in the abdomen where nerve pathways can become irritated and painful. If it is too painful to move your body during menstruation, consistent movement during the rest of the month can help by increasing core stability. A stable core that is both strong and supple helps the lumbar spine musculature move better and assists in alleviating cramping and pain. Beyond movement, food also has an effect on period-related pain. A 2018 study examining dietary patterns and dysmenorrhea found that a diet high in sugar, salty snacks, desserts, sweets, tea, coffee, fruit juice, and saturated and trans fats is associated with an increased risk of dysmenorrhea. The overconsumption of these types of food displaces and decreases the intake of nutrient-dense foods, which results in micronutrient deficiencies that can further exacerbate inflammation and period pain.

Menstrual cramps—their severity and whether we get them—are connected to our lifestyle and overall health. Below, you'll find a list of actions supported either by anecdotal evidence, research, or both that you can refer to throughout the month that may help relieve or reduce the pain so many of us experience each month. Some of the actions we can take are preventative, like eating nutrient-dense whole foods, while others work well for treating cramps, like hot packs. Additionally, the recipes, movements, and self-care recommendations at the end of this chapter provide specific supportive measures to try so that "pain" is not the word that describes your monthly bleeding experience.

FOOD

- Avoid foods with added sugar, artificial sweeteners, high fructose corn syrup, and refined and processed vegetable oils like corn, soy, and canola.

- Avoid conventional dairy products. If possible, opt for grass-fed, organic milk or plant-based milk alternatives.

- Avoid processed and refined grains, poor-quality conventional meat, and excessive alcohol and caffeine.

- Eat a high-fiber diet including plenty of vegetables, leafy greens, fruits, beans, nuts, seeds, and whole grains.

- Eat plenty of wild fish such as salmon, sardines, anchovies, and mackerel and other omega-3 rich foods such as flax, chia seeds, walnuts, and oysters.

- Add anti-inflammatory spices like turmeric, ginger, and cinnamon to your cooking.

- Consume plentiful healthy fats like extra virgin olive oil, butter from grass-fed cows, ghee, coconut oil, and fat from pastured animals.

- When you eat meat, eggs, seafood, or wild game, eat the good stuff. This means pastured, organic, grass-fed, free-range, and/or wild-caught.

- Eat magnesium-loaded foods like leafy greens, apricots, figs, avocados, salmon, almonds, fermented dairy products, beans/legumes, and sweet potatoes.

- Eat zinc-rich foods such as oysters, mussels, pumpkin seeds, beef, lamb, organ meats, yogurt, chickpeas, and cashews.

- Up your intake of fermented foods like sauerkraut, kimchi, fermented dairy, and lacto-fermented vegetables.

MOVEMENT AND OTHER PRACTICES

- Move your body dynamically, mixing up types of movements. Sit less, move more.

- Sex, masturbation, and orgasms help some people relieve menstrual cramps. Warm baths, hot packs, slowing down, and taking deep diaphragmatic breaths through your nose may also help.

- Cultivate healthy sleep through nutrient-dense food, lots of movement, elimination of screens before bed, a cool and dark room for sleeping, and stress management.

- Work with a supportive provider who acknowledges your pain and listens to your treatment preferences.

- Try out transcutaneous nerve stimulation (TENS), a device your doctor can prescribe that helps many people with cramping pain.

- Consider bodywork including (but not limited to) acupuncture, abdominal massage therapy (Arvigo or Mizan Therapy), craniosacral therapy, massage, and osteopathic or chiropractic treatment. Some people experience great relief with bodywork that addresses tightness in the uterine round ligaments.

- Work with an alignment and biomechanics expert who specializes in movements that help relieve period pain.

- Work with a fertility awareness educator.

- Revisit the most common endocrine-disrupting chemicals in the table on pages 22–23 and conscientiously avoid them.

- Avoid tight clothing and consider trying reusable washable pads instead of tampons or menstrual cups as some people experience more pain with tampons or cups.

- In the case of endometriosis and other underlying conditions, additional testing and treatment may be necessary.

Rest and See

Menstruation is a unifying experience for half of the humans on earth. Unfortunately, we've been largely taught that our periods are an inconvenience that we need to hide, and we're sold solutions to the "problem" of menstruating that encourage us to skip over the moment and keep our productivity high. This all makes sense in the context of a capitalistic, patriarchal culture that wants us to keep going, keep working, and keep buying. We don't want to stop or fall behind, and taking time to rest can be seen as a weakness or failure. But when we check out of the world, we give ourselves the opportunity to check into our bodies.

In her book *How to Do Nothing*, Jenny Odell observed how people around her are full of energy, intensity, and anxiety. She wrote, "I see people caught up not just in notifications but in a mythology of productivity and progress, unable not only to rest but simply see where they are." Menstruation is an opportunity to rest and see where we are just like the tree slows down and takes a break to survive through winter before it puts its energy into growing new leaves during the abundant seasons of spring and summer. There is wisdom in this season of rest and reflection. During this moment of transition and pause, we can resist the pull of productivity, the desire to hack our bodies into submission, and listen instead to the messages coming from within. Honoring and acknowledging our blood—both its physical properties and its symbolism of renewal and transition—are a subtle, yet profound act of resistance that might change the way we experience our inner winters.

THE HORMONE-SKIN-GUT CONNECTION

When we talk about our skin—its appearance, integrity, and function—we're actually talking about the dynamic, bidirectional relationship between the gut and skin and the hormones and microbial populations involved in these organs. The gut microbiome produces, metabolizes, and regulates hormones that influence our skin health, and the skin is a large endocrine organ that synthesizes vitamin D and other hormones, which affect the gut microbiota. This relationship is known as the hormone-skin-gut connection, and it acknowledges that skin health is deeply dependent on and influenced by the interaction among these systems. Both the gut and skin play a crucial role in our immune system and neuroendocrine function. An imbalance in gut bacteria and diminished microbial diversity, or dysbiosis, can alter normal hormone function, which can show up on our skin in the form of acne, psoriasis, melasma, or other skin conditions.

The sex hormones involved in the menstrual cycle are an important part of the hormone-skin-gut connection. Estrogen is essential for the normal functioning of our skin. It is involved in collagen synthesis, skin thickness, barrier function, and wound healing. At the beginning of the menstrual cycle, estrogen levels and skin thickness are lower than later in the cycle when estrogen levels increase. Facial skin has a high concentration of estrogen receptors, so changes in estrogen levels show up on facial skin more than other parts of the body. Progesterone increases sebum production, skin elasticity, and firmness.

Premenstrual exacerbation of skin conditions such as acne is thought to be caused by increased sex hormones and androgens, all of which increase sebum production and skin microflora. Hormonal contraceptives and androgen-reducing medications are commonly prescribed for acne and other inflammatory skin conditions because they reduce biologically active androgens. Another approach to improving skin health and function is to focus on restoring or improving the gut microbiome. This means eating nutrient-dense foods, consuming fermented foods and prebiotics (such as fibrous foods and alliums like onions and garlic), and reducing or eliminating the consumption of refined sugars and processed foods. Sebum is hormone-dependent, so improving the health of the gut is one way to regulate sebum production. What we choose to put on our skin can also help regulate sebum production. Vitamin B_5, retinoids, and vitamins C and E improve skin function by regulating sebaceous gland function and reducing inflammation. Additionally, some people see their skin improve when they avoid products that contain fragrances and essential oils. A few skin care companies are creating products that are biome safe—that is, their products support healthy bacteria while discouraging pathogenic bacteria (see page 254 for a few examples). Along with eating well and using products that are biome safe, managing stress, getting enough sleep, reducing exposure to toxins, and moving your body frequently and abundantly create an environment where your skin health is restored and maintained—with the added benefit of improving overall health.

Self-Care

Create Your Ritual

In the days before your period begins, go for a long walk in a beautiful place and set an intention that aligns with how you would like to experience your menstrual phase. For example, "gentle and pain-free," "stable and grounded," or "connected and embodied." Journal or spend time reading. Meditate with your hands placed one on top of the other on your lower abdomen. Choosing one of these rituals, all of them, or devising your own creates a less stressful and more empowered environment for you to experience your bleeding phase. You can change your experience of your period from one cycle to the next. People with a history of painful periods and high stress are nine times more likely to experience painful periods in the subsequent cycle compared to those with low stress and no history of painful periods. You can't change your history of painful periods, but by decreasing your stress during this cycle, you may decrease the pain of future periods.

Get Intimate (with Yourself)

While some people enjoy having sex and/or masturbating during this phase, others would rather skip it. You can experience intimacy, sexual or not, by taking a warm bath or shower, drinking warming non-caffeinated beverages, and using heating pads or wraps. Many of us learned to feel ashamed of our periods or we hide the event, ignoring, as much as we can, what is happening inside. This is an opportunity to practice seeing yourself and your body differently—with acceptance and appreciation. You don't have to love bleeding; this is more about acknowledging the moment, a meditation on the present where we understand that whatever we're feeling—our physical sensations and emotions—is real in this moment but will pass and change.

Rose and Ginger Infused Castor Oil Warming Compress

You can use this infused oil, developed by the clinical herbalist Mary McCallum of Sierra Roots Wellness, anywhere on your body, but it is especially soothing for abdominal menstrual cramps, back pain, and tender breasts. Heat therapy increases blood flow to the pelvis and reduces bloating from fluid retention, which can decrease pain caused by nerve compression.

Makes 14 ounces for 24 compresses

FOR THE INFUSED OIL

1 ounce dried pink rosebuds or rose petals

1 ounce ground ginger

14 ounces organic castor oil

FOR THE COMPRESS

Hot water bottle or heating pad

Cotton flannel square

Old sheet or towel

Make the infused oil. Put the rosebuds and ginger in a blender and pulse until the herbs are broken down into a powder. Pour the herbs into a sterile 16-ounce mason jar and fill the jar with the castor oil. Tightly screw the lid on the jar and store it in a cool, dark space for 2 to 4 weeks, shaking the jar every few days. Once the castor oil is infused, strain the oil mixture using a fine mesh strainer lined with cheesecloth or a coffee filter into another 16-ounce mason jar and store in a cool, dark space. Stored properly, the infusion will keep for one year.

If you have cramps, make the compress. Set up a relaxing space where you can lay down or sit and rest without distractions for 20 to 30 minutes. Make sure your sheet or towel is laid out to catch any drips, as the castor oil is very thick and can be messy. Fill up a hot water bottle or get your heating pad ready and within reach. Pour a small amount of the infused castor oil onto one side of the cotton flannel square and place the square, oil side down, on your body where you need relief. You can also pour the oil onto your skin and then place the flannel over it. Place the hot water bottle over the clean side of the flannel and meditate, read a book, or just rest and enjoy.

Movement

Moving your body, especially your hips and pelvis, increases blood flow to the uterus and can help reduce or relieve painful bleeding. Certain types of movement also support the functioning of the pelvic floor muscles. Declining levels of estrogen during menstruation are associated with weakness in the pelvic floor muscles. This increased weakness may show up as urge incontinence—when you have to pee and feel like you can't hold it—or increased discomfort during bleeding. For optimal functioning, the pelvic floor muscles need to be toned *and* flexible, able to relax *and* contract. If the muscles are too tight, they compromise the alignment of the sacrum, and the shortened, too-tight pelvic floor muscles are actually weaker. These movements support healthy pelvic floor muscle function and can help eliminate or reduce cramping during the menstrual phase.

A note on stretching: Slowly move into stretches so your neurological system can adapt. First, carefully move into the stretch, pause and back off, then repeat, getting a little deeper with each repetition. Repeat this sequence 10 to 15 times per stretch, dynamically moving your body and not statically holding your stretches. Never stretch into painful ranges. Be wary of repetitive movement practices that overstretch your muscles since this can cause instability, pain, and degeneration. The following movements can be done separately, but an effective movement practice during menstruation may look like a 30-minute to 1-hour walk followed by the floor stretches that follow.

Walking. Walking is hands down one of the best movements for a healthy pelvic floor, and it's a gentle, feel-good movement during the menstrual phase.

Adductor (Inner Thigh) Stretch. Lay on your back with your legs up the wall. Move your butt away from the wall until you have a little space between the floor and your lower back, i.e., your low back is not touching the ground. With your knees straight and feet turned outward, slowly move your legs down into a "V" shape until you feel a gentle inner thigh stretch.

Lunges. Move onto your hands and knees. Place your hands directly under your shoulders and your knees beneath the hips. From your hands and knees, place one foot forward and bring your hands to your hips. Start to move your weight forward, pause on the inhale, and deepen the stretch on the exhale. Move with the breath into this stretch for 30 seconds per side.

Abdomen Release Stretch (Modified Cat-Cow). Place your hands and knees on the floor, again with your hands directly under your shoulders, knees under your hips. Keep your neck in line with your spine, looking at the floor. As you inhale, let your stomach fully expand and relax, releasing any tension. As you exhale, gently engage the lower abdominal muscles, pulling them up and into your spine. Repeat 10 times.

Bridge with Knee Squeeze. Lie on your back with your hands along your sides and palms facing down and your knees bent and feet flat on the floor, about hip-width apart. Place a pillow or block between your knees. As you exhale, engage your lower abdominal muscles and glutes, and gently squeeze the block as you lift your butt off the ground. Inhale and release so your butt almost touches the ground, then repeat 10 times.

Reclined Bound Angle Pose. Lay on your back, bend your knees, and place your feet flat on the ground. Draw your heels toward your pelvis and press the soles of your feet together, allowing your knees to drop open on both sides. Place one hand on your low belly and one on your heart and take 10 deep belly breaths.

Reclining Twist. Lying on your back with your legs extended, exhale and feel your shoulders and spine relax and connect to the ground. Engage your lower abdomen and pull your right leg with a bent knee into your chest. Then slowly guide your leg across your body to the left so that you're in a lying spinal twist. Place your left hand on your right knee, deepening the stretch, while your right hand extends away from your body. Turn your head to the right, gazing at your right hand. Take 10 deep belly breaths, gently deepening the stretch in your right glute while trying to keep your shoulders on the ground. Slowly release, then stretch the other side.

Child's Pose. Find your way to hands and knees again. With your hands planted under your shoulders, move your knees apart so they are slightly wider than hip-distance apart. Bring your big toes together, then slide your hands forward and exhale as you lay your torso down between your thighs. Take 10 deep breaths into your sacrum, feel your tailbone lengthen, and tuck your chin so your forehead is resting on the ground. Child's Pose is especially comforting for cramping pain.

A NOTE ON FOOD

Food—whether we're talking about plants, animals, fish, or fungi—represents a web of relationships. No single ingredient is actually singular; each represents an ecological community where plants and animals interact with bacteria, fungi, viruses, and organisms large and small. Biodiversity, a richness in the variety of life-forms in an ecosystem, allows plants, animals, and soil to thrive and produce healthy food for us to eat.

Many people use labels such as "vegetarian" or "paleo." These labels put us into distinct groups, can create conflicts between groups (vegans versus carnivores), and may leave out the reality that, no matter how you choose to eat, you are interacting in and affecting the food web of relationships. This way of thinking is reductive and misses the crucial point that everything is connected in a complex, integrated system that needs diversity for the health of the whole.

Food is emotional and spiritual. It carries a religious power, urging many eaters to go on lifelong missions to convert others to what they consider the "right" way of eating. I urge you, as a human who must eat to survive, not to think of the way you eat as "right" or "wrong," but to think about how the food you choose to eat affects the ecosystem you live in and the ecosystem within your body. My favorite way to think about the impact of food on these ecosystems is to examine how the food was grown and how the growing style has an impact on soil health. Whether you're a flexitarian, vegetarian, or omnivore, the kale, tempeh, or grass-fed beef you enjoy was grown or raised in fields and pastures that either depleted or regenerated soil health. Certain forms of agriculture place soil health at the center of their missions and ideology. Regenerative agriculture, for example, recognizes that healthy soil filled with life is key to producing high-quality, nutrient-dense food. In contrast to the industrialized food system, this method of farming and grazing focuses on improving soil health and the whole ecosystem instead of degradation and extraction. Food grown this way has the power to rebuild the health of our bodies and ecosystems.

The recipes in this book are omnivorous; that is, they feature both plants and animals (and fungi and bacteria). They are open to alterations, substitutions, and changes based on seasonality and your preferences. However you define the way you eat, my hope is that, when possible, you'll choose foods based less on their dietary labeling and more on whether that food was grown in a way that promotes thriving soil and a flourishing ecosystem. Often, the best place to find food grown this way is from small farms and farmers' markets because more farms are starting to use regenerative principles in their growing practices. We might not all agree on the "right" way to eat, but all of us can be soil advocates, and thus ecosystem and taste advocates, by choosing food that is cultivated with healthy soil in mind.

MENSTRUAL PHASE
Recipes

Wild Salmon Congee with Broccolini, Kimchi, and Avocado

Wild salmon is rich in anti-inflammatory omega-3 fatty acids, DHA, and vitamin D while broccolini is high in vitamin C. Both foods nourish the body and help relieve menstrual cramps. Congee (also called rice porridge, jook, and many other names across Asia) is a staple in Asian cuisine, dating back thousands of years as a healing food that promotes good health and digestion. It is the ultimate comfort food and equally delicious with poached eggs, mushrooms, and vegetables or leafy greens.

Makes 6 servings

1 cup short-grain brown rice

3 cups bone broth or vegetable broth

3 cups water

Olive oil

Sea salt

1 pound wild salmon, skin on

½ lemon, thinly sliced

2 bunches (1 pound) broccolini

2 teaspoons shoyu, tamari, or coconut aminos

TO SERVE

Kimchi

Avocado slices

Sprouts (broccoli, radish, or pea)

Lemon juice

Rinse the rice under running water until the water runs clear. Place the rice in a large pot on the stovetop and add the broth and water. Cover the pot and bring the rice to a boil, then turn the heat down low and simmer for 40 to 50 minutes until it is creamy and thickened.

While the rice is cooking, preheat the oven to 275°F. Drizzle some olive oil in a baking dish, salt the salmon on both sides, then place it in the dish. Place the lemon slices on top of the salmon, drizzle with more olive oil, and roast in the oven until the salmon is flaky, tender, and the middle is still pink and just cooked through, about 20 to 30 minutes depending on the thickness of the fish.

About 10 minutes before the salmon is done, heat 2 tablespoons of olive oil in a large skillet over medium-high heat. Add the broccolini, sprinkle with salt, and cook uncovered until it is bright green and slightly charred on all sides. Cover the broccolini and cook for another few minutes until it is tender and crisp.

Stir the 2 teaspoons of shoyu into the congee and serve immediately in large bowls with the tender salmon, broccolini, kimchi, avocado slices, sprouts, and a squeeze of lemon juice on top.

Slow-Roasted Chicken and Sweet Potatoes with Kale, Garlic, and Parsley

Organic, pastured, and free-range chicken provides plentiful protein and healthy fat that stabilizes blood sugar and replenishes iron levels that can be lost during bleeding. The slow roasting makes for delicious and tender meat and is low maintenance, so you could take a walk or run an errand while it roasts. Sweet potatoes, kale, garlic, and parsley support healthy estrogen metabolism and are rich in antioxidants and phytonutrients.

Makes 4 servings

One 3½–4 pound chicken

1 lemon, quartered

2 sprigs fresh rosemary

1 bunch of kale, stems removed and greens roughly chopped

1 clove garlic, minced

Olive oil

Sea salt

4 sweet potatoes

1 bunch fresh parsley, tender stems and leaves cut into 1-inch pieces

Plain full-fat yogurt or cultured sour cream

Generously season the chicken with salt and pepper at least 30 minutes before cooking (you could also do this the night before). Allow the chicken to come to room temperature for 30 to 60 minutes before roasting.

Preheat the oven to 300°F. Place the chicken breast side up in a baking dish, cast iron, or roasting pan and stuff the chicken with the rosemary sprigs and 2 lemon wedges. Let it roast for 30 minutes.

Place the rinsed and dried sweet potatoes on a baking sheet lined with parchment paper or a silicone baking mat. Drizzle the potatoes with a little olive oil and a sprinkle of sea salt. Put the potatoes in the same 300°F oven next to or on the rack below the chicken. Roast for about 1 hour, then take the chicken out of the oven and scatter the kale and garlic around it, seasoning everything with olive oil and salt. Continue roasting for about 30 minutes until the chicken's skin is browned and the meat is tender and the sweet potatoes are completely tender and cooked through. If you can easily pierce the sweet potatoes with a fork, they are done.

Take the chicken and sweet potatoes out of the oven and set the oven to broil, or 500°F. Set the chicken aside. Slit the top of the sweet potatoes lengthwise and ⅓ into the potato flesh. Broil until the skin starts to brown and crisp, about 5 minutes.

Serve the chicken, kale, garlic, cooked lemon, and sweet potatoes with the remaining lemon, parsley, and yogurt. If you have leftover chicken, check out the Tom Kha Gai soup below.

Tom Kha Gai with Mushrooms, Lemongrass, and Chicken

Tom Kha Gai is a popular Thai soup. You can find ingredients like lemongrass, ginger, mushrooms, Thai chilies, and fish sauce at most natural food stores or Asian markets. Bone broth is also available frozen at most grocery stores, or you can save money and make a large pot of bone broth at home [I save all my roasted chicken carcasses, freeze them, and when I have three, I put them in a large Dutch oven, cover the bones with fresh water to the top of the pot, and simmer on very low heat for 24 hours. Then, strain the bones and save the broth. This yields 6 quarts of bone broth]. Bone broth is rich in minerals, gelatin, amino acids, glycine, and collagen. During menstruation, bone broth is especially soothing and can help relieve digestive discomfort and ease inflammation, which in turn may relieve or ease cramping. This slightly spicy, fragrant soup is delicious and deeply comforting.

Makes 4 servings

RECIPE CONTINUES

Neutral oil (grapeseed or avocado oil)

1 shallot, diced

1-inch piece fresh ginger, minced

1 stalk lemongrass, chopped

5 cups chicken bone broth or vegetable broth

10 ounces oyster mushrooms (shiitake or maitake work well too), stemmed with caps sliced

1 pound slow-roasted chicken removed from the bone shredded into bite-size pieces (substitute organic tempeh if desired)

Two 13.5-ounce cans full-fat coconut milk

½ cup water

2 tablespoons fish sauce (I like Red Boat.)

1 teaspoon coconut palm sugar

2 fresh Thai chilies, cut lengthwise, seeds removed and minced or 1 teaspoon cracked red pepper flakes

Salt

¼ cup lime juice and extra lime wedges (3–4 limes)

Cilantro, roughly chopped

Heat 1 tablespoon of neutral oil in a large Dutch oven on the stovetop and sauté the shallot over medium–low heat for 5 minutes. Add the ginger and lemongrass, and stir into the shallots.

Add the chicken bone broth and simmer for 10 to 15 minutes, then add the mushrooms and chicken. Cook and simmer over medium–low heat until the mushrooms are softened and the chicken is warmed through.

Stir in the coconut milk, water, fish sauce, sugar, and chilies and bring to a gentle simmer. Taste and add salt and lime juice as needed. Serve with lime wedges and cilantro.

Grass-Fed Lamb Curry with Cauliflower, Charred Tomatoes, Ginger, and Turmeric

This nourishing curry replenishes iron and B_{12} with grass-fed lamb while ginger and turmeric offer anti-inflammatory benefits. Coconut milk and bone broth are rich in healthy fats, vitamins, and minerals and can help with satiety and cramps. Make this curry the week leading up to or during your menstrual phase.

Makes 4 servings

Olive oil

1 head of cauliflower, florets and stems sliced into ½-inch-thick pieces

Sea salt

Butter or ghee

4 medium carrots, diced

1-inch piece fresh ginger, minced

½-inch piece fresh turmeric, minced

1 heaping tablespoon curry powder (Curio Spice Comfort Curry is one of my favorites.)

1 bunch dark leafy greens, stems removed and coarsely chopped (I like chard or kale.)

Two 13.5-ounce cans full-fat coconut milk

1 cup chicken bone broth

10 cherry tomatoes or 2–3 large tomatoes, left whole if small, quartered if large

Fresh ground black pepper

1 pound ground lamb or beef (substitute 1 cup cooked chickpeas if desired)

TO SERVE

Fresh herbs such as parsley or cilantro, chopped

Plain full-fat yogurt

Lemon juice

Cooked short grain brown rice

Heat 2 tablespoons of olive oil in a large cast iron pan on the stovetop. Add the cauliflower, season with salt, and cook over medium-high heat stirring occasionally until slightly browned (about 8 minutes).

RECIPE CONTINUES

While the cauliflower cooks, heat 1 tablespoon of butter and 1 tablespoon of olive oil in a large Dutch oven on the stovetop. Add the carrots, ginger, and turmeric and sizzle over medium heat until fragrant for about 5 minutes. Add the curry powder to the pot and bloom it in the hot oil for 30 seconds. Stir to combine, then add the browned cauliflower and leafy greens. Stir in the coconut milk and bone broth, cover, and cook over medium-low heat.

While the curry simmers, heat 2 tablespoons of olive oil in the skillet you used for the cauliflower and add the tomatoes. Season with salt and pepper and cook over medium-high heat until bubbling and slightly charred on both sides. Then, add the lamb. Season with more salt, break up the meat with a spoon, and press it into the skillet. Cook the lamb until it is browned and crispy on both sides.

Spoon the curry into individual serving bowls and top with the lamb and tomatoes. Serve with the fresh herbs, yogurt, lemon juice, and rice.

Watercress Salad with Pan-Fried Oyster Mushrooms and Almond Butter Miso Dressing

This dish is loaded with magnesium-rich foods and healthy fats. Magnesium is an evidence-backed magical mineral that helps calm the nervous system, relieve or prevent menstrual cramps and migraines, and improve insulin resistance. The greens in this dish are balanced by the pan-fried mushrooms, creamy dressing, and crunchy pumpkin seeds.

Makes 4 servings

FOR THE DRESSING

4 tablespoons olive oil

3 tablespoons almond butter (or other nut butter)

Juice from ½ lemon

2 tablespoons warm water

1 tablespoon white miso paste

1 teaspoon raw honey

FOR THE SALAD

2 tablespoons olive oil

12 ounces shitake or oyster mushrooms

2 tablespoons butter or ghee

Sea salt and fresh ground black pepper

12 ounces watercress (arugula, spinach, and baby kale work well too)

½ cup sprouted, raw, or toasted pumpkin seeds

1 avocado, sliced

Make the dressing. Place all the ingredients in a small mason jar, put the lid on, and shake vigorously until well mixed.

Make the salad. Heat the olive oil in the skillet over medium heat and add the mushrooms. Spread the mushrooms out evenly and cook them undisturbed for 5 minutes until they start to brown. Turn the mushrooms and cook for another 5 minutes. Add the butter, turn the heat to low, and cook for another 5 minutes. When the mushrooms are deeply browned and nearly crispy, season the mushrooms with salt and pepper to taste.

Arrange the watercress in a serving bowl. Spoon the warm mushrooms onto the watercress. Drizzle with the dressing and top with the pumpkin seeds and avocado slices. This salad pairs wonderfully with the slow-roasted chicken (see page 84).

Sweet or Savory Snacking Chickpeas

Rich in protein, folate, fiber, B vitamins, and iron, chickpeas (or garbanzo beans) are tasty and nutrient-dense. Vitamin B_6 supports the production of progesterone and also supports the liver's metabolism of estrogen. While you can definitely use canned chickpeas in a pinch, I prefer to buy dried chickpeas and cook my own because dried chickpeas are less expensive than canned and I like controlling the amount of salt in my beans.

Makes 2 cups

CHOOSE ONE SPICE COMBINATION

SAVORY, SPICY, AND LEMONY

1½ tablespoons olive oil

1 teaspoon cayenne pepper or curry powder

Squeeze of lemon juice

Sea salt and fresh ground black pepper

SWEET, CRUNCHY, AND CINNAMONY

1½ tablespoons melted coconut oil

2 teaspoons coconut palm sugar, maple sugar, or honey

½ teaspoon cinnamon

Sea salt

Preheat the oven to 425°F. Dry the cooked chickpeas on a dish towel (if using canned beans, rinse thoroughly first), then roast on a dry, parchment-lined baking sheet for 10 minutes. While the chickpeas roast, mix together all the ingredients from the spice combination of your choice.

Remove the chickpeas from the oven and pour the oil spice mixture on top, stirring to evenly coat. Bake for another 12 to 15 minutes, shaking the pan halfway through. Remove from the oven, let cool, and then enjoy a sweet or savory crispy snack.

Cooking Dried Chickpeas

To begin, you can either soak the beans for a few hours or overnight (which decreases cooking time) or simply cook them without soaking (which takes about twice as long). If I forget to soak the beans overnight, I like the quick-soak method, where you place a cup of beans in a large saucepan and cover them with 3 inches of water. Bring the water to a boil and boil the beans for 5 minutes. Turn the heat off and let the beans sit for an hour in the water.

Whether you soak overnight, do the quick method, or skip soaking, rinse the chickpeas and put them in a large pot on the stovetop. Add water to the pot until the chickpeas are covered by 3 inches. Bring the pot to a boil, then cook over low heat until the chickpeas are tender (about 45 minutes) for the presoaked or quick-soaked beans and 90 minutes for unsoaked beans. Cooked chickpeas can be stored in the fridge for up to a week or frozen for a month.

Citrus and Collagen-Rich Creamsicle Cups

This recipe is a fun and tasty way to use the juice (and pulp—don't leave out the pulp!) of satsumas, tangerines, blood oranges, navels, cara caras, and other types of citrus—try it with whatever is available where you live! The addition of grass-fed beef gelatin (which is flavorless) and the layer of coconut cream on top adds a sense of balance and dimension and ups the nutrition of this creamsicle treat.

Makes six 4-ounce servings

ORANGE LAYER

2 cups citrus juice, divided

1 tablespoon plus 1 teaspoon grass-fed beef gelatin

⅛ teaspoon vanilla bean powder or extract

CREAM LAYER

One 5.4-ounce can full-fat coconut cream or ½ cup heavy whipping cream, divided

2 teaspoons grass-fed beef gelatin

1 teaspoon raw honey or maple syrup (optional)

⅛ teaspoon vanilla bean powder or extract

Make the orange layer. In a small saucepan, combine 2 tablespoons of citrus juice with the gelatin. Stir together until well-combined and allow it to bloom for 1 minute. Put the saucepan on the stovetop and turn the heat on medium. Stir in ½ cup of citrus juice until just warmed through. Turn off the heat and add the remaining juice and vanilla, whisking well to combine. Pour the mixture into silicone molds, ramekins, six 4-ounce mason jars, or a larger dish, leaving ¼ inch of room on top for the cream layer. Chill in the refrigerator until set.

Make the cream layer. Once the orange layer is firm, make the cream layer. In a small saucepan, combine 2 tablespoons of the coconut cream with the gelatin, stirring well and allowing it to bloom for 1 minute. Put the saucepan on the stovetop and turn the heat on medium. Add the rest of the coconut cream, honey, and vanilla bean, warming until just heated through. Pour the cream layer on top of the citrus layer and chill in the refrigerator for another two hours until firm. Serve by popping the treat out of the silicone molds, with a spoon out of ramekins or jars, or slice into small squares if in a larger dish.

Chocolate-Chaga Avocado Pudding

Chaga has a long history as an immune-boosting medicinal mushroom. The fungus grows primarily on birch trees in cold northern climates and is often consumed as tea. Rich in beta-glucans, a type of polysaccharide that supports immune health, chaga is known for its anti-inflammatory, immune-boosting, antioxidant, and cancer-preventing properties. This recipe uses chaga powder, which you can find in natural food stores or order online, combined with cacao and avocado, both rich in magnesium and B vitamins, to create a decadent, healthy, and incredibly easy dessert that nourishes your body.

Makes 4 large or 6 small servings

Flesh of 2 large ripe avocados

One 13.5-ounce can full-fat coconut cream

¾ cup cacao powder

¼ cup pure maple syrup

2 teaspoons chaga powder

¼ teaspoon vanilla powder or 1 teaspoon vanilla extract

¼ teaspoon salt

⅓ cup warm water

To serve: whipped cream, fresh fruit, cinnamon (optional)

Put the avocados, coconut cream, cacao powder, maple syrup, chaga powder, vanilla powder, and salt in a blender and blend on high speed until well-combined (about one minute). Then scrape down the sides with a rubber spatula. With the blender running, add in the warm water and blend until smooth.

Serve the pudding warm or chilled with whipped cream, fresh fruit, and a dash of cinnamon if desired. The pudding will keep for three days if covered and chilled in the refrigerator.

Ashwagandha Moon Milk

Moon milk is a traditional Ayurvedic healing food rooted in ancient botanical medicine. There are many variations of this drink using different healing herbs. This recipe incorporates the adaptogen ashwagandha (Indian ginseng), which is used as Rasayana, or rejuvenation, within Ayurveda as it helps support stress resilience and overall health. Current clinical research supports the use of this plant for its stress-related benefits, including its calming effect and propensity to promote restorative sleep. In the research, participants are typically given 250 to 600 mg/day of ashwagandha for sixty days. For quality information about herbs, access to fresh plant medicine, and effective dosing, it is beneficial to work with a clinical herbalist. You can use dried spices in this recipe (in smaller amounts), but I love the flavor of whole, fresh spices, which can be found at most grocery stores or online. I buy many of my spices from the local food co-op and from Curio Spice Shop, an online market selling fresh whole and ground spices (see more sourcing information in the resources section).

Makes 1 serving

1½ cups dairy or nondairy milk

2 tablespoons heavy cream or half and half (optional)

1-inch piece fresh ginger, minced

½-inch piece fresh turmeric, minced

4 cardamom pods, crushed

1 cinnamon stick

1 teaspoon ground ashwagandha

1 teaspoon ghee

1 teaspoon raw honey (optional)

Fresh ground black pepper

In a small saucepan, combine the milk, cream (if using), ginger, turmeric, cardamom, cinnamon stick, and ashwagandha. Simmer over low heat, stirring occasionally until the milk is deeply infused with flavor (about 5 to 8 minutes).

Pour the moon milk through a fine mesh strainer and into your favorite mug, then stir in the ghee and honey (if using) and finish with a grind of pepper.

Dandelion Burdock Root Chai

Dandelion is often used as a mild digestive bitter that increases bile flow, and it may also help relieve fluid retention, gas, bloating, and nausea. Burdock root is a traditional healing food and medicine that is used to support skin health and digestion. With these two paired with the warming spices, this chai is especially soothing during menstruation. This recipe was developed by the clinical herbalist Mary McCallum.

Makes 2 servings

2 tablespoons dried dandelion root

2 tablespoons dried burdock root

2 teaspoons ground cinnamon

2 teaspoons cardamom pods, crushed

One 1-inch piece fresh ginger, minced

1 teaspoon cloves

4 cups water

Dairy or nondairy milk, steamed or heated

Raw honey or maple syrup

Add the herbs and water to a small saucepan. Cover and simmer the herbs over medium heat for 10 to 15 minutes. Strain the chai using a fine mesh strainer into a 32-ounce mason jar. Pour your desired amount of chai into a mug and add the milk and honey.

Store extra chai in the refrigerator for up to a week, gently reheating and adding milk and honey to taste before consuming.

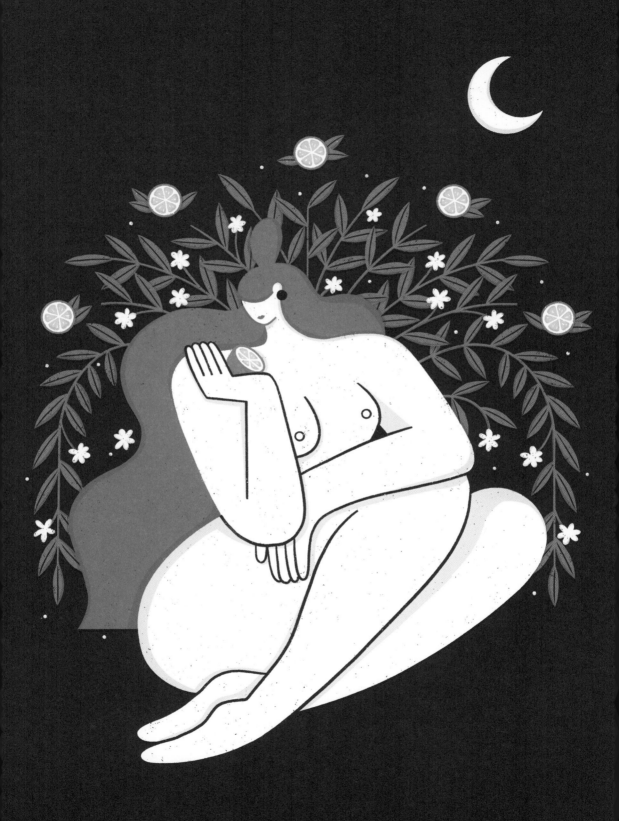

Preovulatory Phase

SPRING • RENEW + CREATE

After resting all winter, deciduous trees wake up in the spring. Water from the melting snow is absorbed by the tree's roots and combines with the stored sugars and nutrients. This sap flows through the tree, delivering the energy and nutrition that is required to create new leaves, which, once they grow, start to photosynthesize sunlight, allowing the leaves to flourish through spring and summer. The tree tracks this cyclic growth with its own timekeeping method: a ring on its trunk to mark another season of renewal.

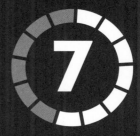

Like the tree, we enter a period of proliferative growth and abundant energy during the springtime of our cycles. In the time following bleeding and preceding ovulation, from about day eight to day sixteen or whenever ovulation occurs in your cycle, the endometrium thickens and grows. Starting with a feeling of subtle awakening, which then shifts into a feeling of blooming and abundance, the spring of your body is marked by dynamic transitions. This transition is largely fed by climbing estrogen levels. Picture a garden bed at the beginning of the growing season. At first, the soil looks bare, and the growth of new seeds is slow. As early spring shifts into late spring, the seeds, nourished by the soil, sun, and water, become full-grown plants with their own recognizable morphology. The same type of growth happens with the inner lining of the endometrium, which sheds during menstruation, then fully regenerates throughout the rest of the month. Breast tissue tends to feel more buoyant and cervical mucus transforms from infertile to fertile mucus by the end of this phase.

The preovulatory phase requires a carefully orchestrated series of physiological events in order to become the ovulatory phase. These events start with intact communication between the brain and the ovaries. The first half of the cycle, which includes both menstruation and the preovulatory phase, is called the follicular or proliferative phase. This phase is characterized by the maturation of ovarian follicles, a process called folliculogenesis. Ovarian follicles are small fluid-filled sacs that contain an immature egg; there are thousands of these follicles in the ovaries. The word *genesis* means "the beginning," "generation," "the origin," or "coming into being." It's a word that alludes to both creation and transformation, and as such, the genesis of follicles is a journey that doesn't occur overnight. We can consider the process of folliculogenesis as a kind of hero's journey: There is a beginning, or the origin story when follicles first develop within the ovaries of the fetus; a middle, when the follicle might be chosen to develop and become capable of ovulation; and an end, when the follicle either undergoes scheduled, necessary cell death or releases an egg, which starts a new story.

At birth, people with ovaries have around four hundred thousand follicles. These follicles live a quiet, dormant life for decades before some of them are recruited into the growth and development club during puberty. Of the follicles that are chosen, only a few become mature follicles that are able to release an egg. Follicular maturation is a long, drawn-out process that is tightly regulated by our genes, hormones, and other factors. Because the development of a mature follicle takes so long and requires specific, sequential, and coordinated interaction between so many systems, the day when that follicle releases an egg, also known as ovulation, is kind of a big deal. The preovulatory phase is when the body lines everything up like dominoes ready to tip over and set off a cascade of events at the exact right moment.

Several key hormones are involved in preparing for ovulation. One is FSH (follicle stimulating hormone). Preovulatory follicles depend on stimulation from FSH to mature, and the dominant follicle—the one destined for ovulation—becomes dominant by increasing its sensitivity to FSH while the other follicles compete for diminishing levels of FSH. Sometimes more than one dominant follicle develops and releases an egg (this is how twins and multiples happen). But usually, only one dominant follicle survives and releases an egg each month. This follicle produces estrogen that tells the pituitary to stop secreting FSH, which inhibits the growth of its sibling follicles. Increasing production of estrogen shifts the dominant follicle from its FSH-sensitive state to an LH (luteinizing hormone)-sensitive state. Estrogen production from the dominant follicle peaks the day before LH levels surge, which induces ovulation. As estrogen climbs throughout this phase, so does testosterone, which peaks during the ovulatory phase. In the ovaries, the enzyme aromatase catalyzes the conversion of androgen hormones such as testosterone to estrogens. Testosterone and other androgen hormones are essential for normal ovarian function and follicular development. The action isn't limited to the ovaries. Climbing estrogen levels affect our immune function and, in general, we're less susceptible to infections during the follicular phase. Insulin sensitivity is also impacted by increased estrogen, and we tend to tolerate carbohydrates better during the first half of our cycles.

As estrogen levels steadily climb during the preovulatory phase, peaking right before ovulation, it is common to experience increased energy, and you may also feel sexier and more sexual as estrogen increases blood flow to your genitals. The experience of this phase can feel really good. It can feel like a time of openness, curiosity, and creativity when the physical processes of change and growth happening in our bodies are reflected in how we process ourselves and others in the world. If we feel fatigued, dull, or off during the preovulatory phase, we're receiving a signal that we need to assess our sleep, eating, and movement habits, or perhaps an underlying medical condition, so we can take care of our specific needs.

I imagine the preovulatory phase like the apricot tree in my garden. It is the first tree to blossom in the early spring, and when the spring is mild, without stress from hard frosts, the blossoms become golden fruit at the peak of summer. The tree needs the right conditions in the springtime, the preovulatory phase in this metaphor, to fruit in the summertime, the ovulatory phase. And, some years, not a single apricot can be found on the tree. When this happens, I observe the tree and do my best to continue to support its health throughout the year with the hope that, with care, attention, and patience, I'll again see fruit on its branches.

SEED CYCLING

Often recommended by alternative medicine practitioners to regulate the menstrual cycle and to treat and correct estrogen and progesterone imbalances, seed cycling involves eating different seed combinations during different phases of the menstrual cycle: one tablespoon each of raw flaxseeds and pumpkin seeds during the follicular phase (starting on the first day of bleeding) and one tablespoon each of raw sesame seeds and sunflower seeds during the luteal phase (starting on the day of ovulation). The seeds are consumed every single day (that's two tablespoons of raw seeds a day) and can be added to foods like pesto, bars, cookies, smoothies, salads, and seed balls.

The theory behind seed cycling is that lignans—a polyphenol found in the seeds' hulls—help regulate hormone levels. Even though these seeds have great nutritional value, there isn't research that shows consuming these specific seeds has a measurable effect on hormone levels. There *is* research showing that flaxseeds can reduce androgen levels in individuals with PCOS and can help decrease cyclical breast pain. So, if you don't have any allergies to the aforementioned seeds, there's not much risk involved in trying seed cycling. On pages 119 and 181, you'll find basic recipes for seed cycling during the follicular and luteal phases. Enjoy them as recommended by seed cycling enthusiasts or during any time of the month.

Eating and Your Cycle

Because our body chemistry changes—as does our appetite and metabolism—it makes sense to adjust how we eat, move, and take care of ourselves during each phase. One way to adjust is to practice periodization, syncing the way we eat and move to the menstrual cycle. In a 2016 study published in the *American Journal of Clinical Nutrition*, sixty healthy, overweight (defined as a body mass index (BMI) of 25–30), premenopausal, cisgender women were recruited and randomly assigned to a six-month weight-loss program.

In the control group, the intervention for weight loss was energy restriction (eating less food), while the test group individuals were given a diet plan that was synchronized to match a twenty-eight-day menstrual cycle. Dubbed the Menstralean diet, the macronutrient composition of the meals was aligned with the average length of the menstrual, follicular, and luteal phases. During the follicular and luteal phases, the Menstralean diet upped daily protein intake from 20 percent to 30 percent of total calories. Fat intake increased from 20 percent during the menstrual and follicular phase to 30 percent during the luteal phase. Individuals were also allowed extra dark chocolate during the luteal phase. Finally, carbohydrate intake was highest during the menstrual phase and lowest during the luteal phase.

The changes in the macronutrient composition reflect the metabolic changes that occur during each phase of the cycle. When estrogen levels are high during the follicular phase, we tend to experience a decrease in our appetite, whereas high progesterone levels during the luteal phase may stimulate appetite. One study showed that, compared to the follicular phase, naturally cycling individuals increased their food consumption between 90 to 500 calories per day during the luteal phase. These changes in appetite appear to be related to glucose homeostasis. During the luteal phase, insulin sensitivity is lower than during the follicular phase, which means we tend to maintain better glucose homeostasis during the follicular phase. Energy needs increase just prior to and during menstruation. The Menstralean diet reflects this increased energy need by upping the daily percentage of fat intake and including rations for dark chocolate.

The Menstralean diet group was also assigned an exercise program that was tailored to the menstrual cycle with light activity such as walking or yoga during the menstrual phase, weight and circuit training during the follicular phase, and alternating cardiovascular and weight training during the luteal phase. The control exercise program was the same throughout the month and consisted of thirty minutes of exercise every day with twenty minutes of high-intensity exercise two days a week. The rationale for different forms of exercise during each phase was to maximize energy expenditure, which is why more intense forms of exercise were assigned during the luteal phase when energy intake is greater.

Even though this small study measured weight loss as an outcome, what's valuable is not its focus on dieting and restriction—a toxic topic in US culture—but rather the idea of eating and moving with the menstrual cycle. The Menstralean diet, even with its limitations, acknowledged that our cycle has a real impact on our physiology and metabolism.

If you're interested to give it a go, practicing this in your own life does not require strict diets and protocols. It only requires paying attention to how you feel. Only by first paying attention can we then adjust our behaviors in ways that sync us with our biology. This kind of mindfulness deeply connects us to the experience of our menstrual cycle and how it influences our basic physiology day-to-day. It also encourages us to be flexible and open-minded. If you are used to working out the same way all the time or eating the same food most days, experimenting with how you move and eat during different phases of your cycle helps break that routine and serves the dual purpose of introducing more diverse food and movement into your life.

A growing number of studies are finding that when people eat mindfully, which includes making deliberate choices about the food we eat and how we eat it while cultivating awareness of our internal state in relation to what we eat, individuals improve their long-term metabolic health. In one study, participants were trained in mindful eating practices—that is, paying purposeful attention to their food, moment to moment, without judgment—and were encouraged to practice mindfulness meditation for thirty minutes a day. Compared to the control group, these individuals ate fewer sweets and experienced improved fasting blood glucose levels. Crucially, these results lasted a long time, meaning eating this way improves your health in the long run. Paying attention to how food tastes and our level of satisfaction with that food while eliminating distractions such as phones or TV are tools that help us become more mindful eaters. This act of placing your food in front of you and giving it your full attention promotes healthy eating patterns while allowing you to enjoy your food and connect what you eat to how you feel.

ALL ABOUT VAGINAL STEAMING

Vaginal steaming, also known as pelvic steaming, yoni steaming, or v-steaming, involves sitting over a steaming pot of water infused with herbs. The practice allows aromatic steam to rise to your nether regions. While vaginal steaming has ancient roots, it is also increasingly trendy. The practice is controversial, with many holistic practitioners swearing by its healing powers and most gynecologists either adamantly warning against it or stating that there is no scientific evidence to support steaming.

The Claims. Vaginal steaming is believed to soothe and detoxify the body of both toxins and toxic emotions, increase blood flow to the pelvic floor muscles and vaginal tissues, increase cervical fluid, and cleanse the uterus. Proponents of steaming say that this self-care practice supports hormonal balance, regular menstrual cycles, postpartum healing, fertility, sexual health, detoxification, and tension and stress relief. Additionally, steaming is meant to soothe menstrual cramps; alleviate hemorrhoids; help with conditions like PCOS, PMS, and endometriosis; reduce infections like UTIs and yeast infections; relieve menopause symptoms like dryness; connect us deeper to our bodies; help with painful sexual intercourse; and aid in healing from sexual trauma. Steaming is not recommended for individuals who are ovulating, trying to conceive, or currently pregnant. It is also not recommended for those with an IUD, with active infections, or who are currently menstruating.

CONTINUES

The Science. The anecdotal evidence on vaginal steaming abounds, but the scientific evidence on the practice is lacking. One (very) small preliminary study found compelling positive results in steaming among postpartum women including reduced blood pressure and heart rate; increased weight loss and waist size reduction; improved uterus restoration, labial healing, and bowel regularity; and hemorrhoid reduction. The results of this study are promising, but more studies are needed with larger and more diverse sample sizes.

While steaming is often promoted as a healing and nurturing practice, it is also often marketed as a method of cleansing and purification. Advertising vaginal steaming this way inherently assumes that our bodies are impure and dirty. This is a harmful assumption that has roots in ancient medical practices and continues today through products and practices such as vaginal steaming that are touted as improvements to our bodies, bodies we're told are tainted and deficient. The reality is that the vagina is remarkably adept at self-cleaning. Capable of resisting and fighting infections, the vagina and its microbiome is a thriving environment that doesn't require detoxification or cleansing. A healthy vaginal microbiome—which is mostly composed of *Lactobacillus* bacteria—fights pathogenic infections and maintains an acidic pH. Some ways to promote natural and healthy vaginal flora include avoiding douching and washing with harsh soaps, prioritizing a healthy diet rich in fermented foods, and wearing breathable fabrics like cotton underwear and loose clothing.

Your Choice. Steaming may disturb the pH of the vagina, which increases the risk of infection and irritation. The vagina doesn't require deep cleaning. That said, there are incredible accounts of healing, such as relief from menstrual cramps, among steamers. The debate between those who swear by vaginal steaming and those who swear against it isn't likely to go away anytime soon, but in the end, it is your choice.

Self-Care

Follow the Morning Light

According to the EPA, Americans spend over 90 percent of their waking hours indoors even though exposure to the rhythm of light and dark affects the timing of mechanisms in the brain and regulates our behavior and physiology. We need robust exposure to light that has a high circadian effect (aka sunlight) during the day. Similarly, we need darkness at night. One study showed that receiving high levels of circadian-effective light in the morning helps people fall asleep faster and sleep better at night, syncs physiological and biological rhythms to the environment, and reduces depression. Disruption of circadian rhythms is associated with menstrual cycle disruptions, mood changes, fertility issues, and increases in the risk of breast cancer. Improve your relationship to the natural rhythm of light and dark by making an effort to get at least fifteen minutes of light in the morning, preferably outside from sunlight. If that isn't possible, you may consider investing in a light therapy lamp and use it at work on your desk or in your home. When you have a chance to go outside during the day, take it! The more we match our daily rhythm to the natural light and dark happening outside, the more we support the oscillations of our internal rhythms.

Unplug

Another habit that nurtures our circadian rhythms is taking a break from screens, especially before going to sleep. Exposure to blue light at night is associated with delayed melatonin release, which means more time spent trying to get to sleep and poorer quality sleep. Putting your phone and other devices away at least an hour before bedtime, using blue light filtering glasses or blue light filtering screens for your computer or phone, and using nighttime warm light features on your devices are all strategies you can use to protect your eyes and decrease your exposure to blue light before bedtime.

Revitalizing Salt Scrub

The lymphatic system is a network of organs and tissues that work together to maintain fluid balance, fight infections, and remove waste from the body. Its primary job is to transport lymph—a colorless fluid—through your circulatory system, where it delivers nutrients and removes waste products throughout the body. This salt scrub, developed by the clinical herbalist Mary McCallum, mildly exfoliates the skin, which gently stimulates the lymphatic system. The herbs in this scrub are from the energizing mint family, offering a feeling of lightness, refreshment, and possibility.

Makes 2 cups

1 cup sea salt or pink Himalayan salt

1 cup dried tulsi, spearmint, or lemon balm (or a mix)

4 tablespoons almond oil for dry and irritated skin, coconut oil for cooling and easing

skin discomfort caused by sunburn, or sesame oil for deep moisturization

5–10 drops rosemary essential oil (optional)

To a small mixing bowl, add the salt and herbs. Fold in the herbs and drizzle in your preferred oil and essential oil, if using. Mix well and store in a glass jar. Store the scrub in the shower and use it within 6 months.

To use the scrub, get wet in the shower and then apply a generous palmful, gently exfoliating your shoulders, arms, belly, and legs. Thoroughly rinse off the salt scrub, and after your shower, finish with your favorite body oil or moisturizer.

Movement

Compared to the luteal phase, some studies show that resistance training during the preovulatory and ovulatory phases is more beneficial and associated with greater gains in lean body mass and muscle strength. This means that the time you spend increasing your body strength during this phase pays off with greater overall gains as compared to other phases. Many resources that promote syncing exercise with the menstrual cycle recommend trying out a new workout class, hitting the gym to lift weights, and upping your cardio or high-intensity interval training (HIIT) during this phase. If you like these forms of exercise, you can certainly keep doing them, but I'd like to introduce you to a new movement challenge.

This new movement challenge isn't actually new at all—it's movement as humans have always moved. Some of these natural movements include running, jumping, climbing, crawling, lifting, throwing, carrying, walking, dancing, sprinting, swimming, and squatting. Instead of exercising for a set period of time and calling it good for the day, the challenge is to incorporate movement into the fabric of your life. This challenge is meant to shake up your routine, get you strong in places that might be weak, and give overworked parts of your body a break. The goal is a dynamically strong and balanced body that is above all functional, adaptable, and capable.

Set Up Your Movement Environment

Often the biggest inhibitor of more movement is how we live and the design of our environment. Comfy chairs and couches invite more sitting, cars replace short-distance walking, shoes limit the mobility of our feet, appliances in the kitchen replace the movement involved in food processing, and grocery stores replace thousands of movements involved in growing food. We can redesign and reimagine our environment to increase the amount we move without giving up all of the conveniences of modern life.

What can you add to your space that invites movement and play? One strategy that works brilliantly is to look at your living space like a child. Children are instinctual natural movers. They climb trees and all over furniture, they test their limits when they jump off bigger and bigger rocks, and they sit on the ground often and with ease. Kids get messy, and they aren't afraid to move their bodies. If you see your environment as a child, you'll see movement possibilities everywhere you look.

Here's a few ways to change your environment to help you move more:

- Install a pull-up bar outside your bathroom and hang after each bathroom use.

- Go barefoot whenever possible.

- Create a dynamic work environment with a standing desk or a low desk so you can sit in different positions on the floor and a yoga ball. Take plenty of movement breaks.

- Consider growing some food, even if it's just a few herbs in your window. Or get involved with picking some of your own food at local farms that offer U-pick options.

- If you have small children, try carrying them on some walks instead of using the stroller.

- When cleaning your house, occasionally get down on hands and knees to clean the floor instead of using a mop. As you are able, set up your kitchen so you have to climb, squat, and reach to get what you need.

- Avoid elevators when possible and take the stairs.

- Make a meal, pack it up, and take it into nature for a picnic. Follow the principles of leave no trace.

- Sit on the floor. Sitting or lying on hard surfaces to rest forces us to move our bodies more because staying in one position for too long is uncomfortable.

Create Movement Where It Wasn't Before

This concept is broadly applicable. It applies to our breath, our jobs, and our homelife. Can you breathe deeper, therefore moving your lungs and thoracic diaphragm more? Can you walk to work or park your car farther away, increasing the amount of movement it takes to get to your office or the store? Are you able to carry your groceries around in a basket instead of using a cart, so your body does more work as you shop? There is no part of life too big or too small when it comes to incorporating more movement.

Think of Movement as Ongoing

Movement is broad and accessible; it doesn't always require special equipment (like at a gym), and you can do it anywhere and tailor it to your body's needs. Instead of checking exercise off your to-do list after a one-hour workout, challenge yourself to move and keep moving throughout the day.

Recipes

Lacto-Fermented Ginger and Turmeric Carrots

Lacto-fermentation is the process of allowing *Lactobacillus* bacteria, which are naturally present on foods like cabbage and other fruits and vegetables, to break down sugars and form lactic acid and carbon dioxide, preserving food while also boosting its nutritional value and tastiness. This simple recipe can be applied to many vegetables and even condiments like hot sauce. The more fermented foods we can incorporate into our everyday meals, the better off our gut and overall health.

Makes 32 ounces

2 cups room temperature water

2 teaspoons sea salt

1½ pounds carrots peeled and cut into matchsticks

1-inch piece fresh ginger, grated

½-inch piece fresh turmeric, grated

In a measuring cup with a spout, mix the water and salt until combined. Pack the carrot sticks, ginger, and turmeric into a 32-ounce mason jar (you can do this with the jar sideways to make it easier). Cover the carrot mixture with the brine, making sure it is completely submerged. Tightly seal the jar and let it sit at room temperature for 2 to 3 days, then move it to the refrigerator to ferment for another 7 days. At this point, the carrots are ready to use and will keep slowly fermenting and developing their flavor in the fridge.

You can use these carrots in the Collard Green Spring Rolls (page 111), or any other dish you can imagine. They are also delicious on their own. Keep them stored in the refrigerator. Use within 3 months.

Collard Green Spring Rolls with Pastured Pork and Nut Butter Dipping Sauce

Collard greens are a rich source of folate and fat-soluble vitamins A and K. Consuming these greens with healthy fat increases the bioavailability of these vitamins. Soaking the collard greens as I do for this recipe softens the greens so they are easier to roll into spring rolls. Adding sauerkraut or lacto-fermented vegetables to these rolls boosts their microbiome benefits. Make these for dinner and encourage family and friends to roll their own.

Makes 6 servings

DIPPING SAUCE

¾ cup cashew, almond, or other nut butter

¼ cup lime juice (from about 2 limes)

4 tablespoons tamari, shoyu, or coconut aminos

2 teaspoons raw honey

1-inch piece ginger, grated

1 Thai chili or jalapeño, minced

2 tablespoons hot water

SPRING ROLLS

Grapeseed or olive oil

1 pound pastured ground pork (or other ground grass-fed meat, wild shrimp, sliced steak, pork belly, or organic tempeh)

Sea salt

1 pound collard greens

6 cups hot water

1 tablespoon apple cider vinegar

1 mango, julienned

1 avocado, thinly sliced

2 stems mint, stems removed, leaves left whole

1 bunch basil, stems removed, leaves left whole

½ cup sprouts, left whole (radish, broccoli, pea, etc.)

Quick Pickles (page 140), Lacto-Fermented Ginger and Turmeric Carrots (page 110), or Purple Sauerkraut (page 138)

RECIPE CONTINUES

Make the dipping sauce. Add the nut butter, lime juice, tamari, honey, ginger, and chili to a small bowl or mason jar. Whisk to combine, then add the hot water and whisk again. (If using a mason jar, you can just put on the lid and shake it to combine.)

Make the spring rolls. In a large cast iron skillet, heat 1 tablespoon of oil. Press the pork into the pan in an even layer, then let it cook over high heat without touching it. Once the pork starts crisping at the edges, break up the meat into pieces with a spatula, season abundantly with salt, and flip so all sides get satisfyingly browned.

Cut the tough stems from the collard greens and discard them. Place the greens in a pan with high sides and pour the hot water over top, covering them completely. Add the apple cider vinegar and allow the greens to soften for 2 to 3 minutes. Drain and pat dry. Cut the collard greens in half lengthwise for serving.

To serve. In separate bowls, place the collard greens, pork, mango, avocado, mint, basil, sprouts, Quick Pickles, and dipping sauce on the table. To assemble the spring rolls (this part is fun for everyone to do themselves), lay a collard green flat on your plate and add each ingredient, rolling the collard green closed when finished. You can add the dipping sauce inside each spring roll or have it on the side to dip.

Roasted Cauliflower with Pumpkin Seeds, Parsley, Mint, and Lemon

Crunchy, salty, and vibrant, this roasted cauliflower dish is delicious, endlessly adaptable, and helps support healthy estrogen metabolism. Cruciferous vegetables like cauliflower, brussels sprouts, bok choy, broccoli, and cabbage contain active ingredients such as indole-3-carbinol and 3,3'-diindolylmethane, which both help the body metabolize estrogen into metabolites that are beneficial for the body. This dish is excellent as a side, with chickpeas added to the roasting pan, or served on a large bed of leafy greens such as arugula for a more complete meal.

Makes 4 servings

1 cauliflower, florets, stem, and green leaves chopped

½ lemon, sliced

2 teaspoons brown mustard seeds

1 teaspoon ground turmeric

3 tablespoons extra virgin olive oil

Sea salt

1 large bunch parsley, coarsely chopped

Leaves from 1–2 stems of mint, coarsely chopped

¼ cup raw sprouted pumpkin seeds (salted or unsalted)

2 heaping tablespoons dried currants

Fromage blanc or queso fresco, or other crumbly cheese

½ lemon

Flaky sea salt

Preheat the oven to 450°F. On a parchment-lined or unlined baking sheet, toss the cauliflower and the lemon slices with the mustard seeds, turmeric, and olive oil and season generously with salt. Roast until the cauliflower is crispy, about 20–25 minutes, stirring once or twice.

Take the cauliflower and lemons out of the oven and toss them with the parsley, mint, pumpkin seeds, and currants in a large bowl. Top with crumbled fromage blanc, a drizzle of olive oil, a squeeze of lemon juice, and flaky sea salt.

Mussels with Kale and Garlic-Parsley Broth

Iodine is a trace mineral that is crucial for thyroid health and the production of thyroid hormones. After the thyroid, the ovaries have the highest iodine concentration, and they require adequate iodine levels to produce estrogen. Bivalves, like mussels, clams, and oysters, are great sources of iodine, selenium, iron, copper, zinc, and vitamin B_{12}. Paired with a nourishing broth, dark leafy greens, and sprouts on top, this dish is a wealth of protein, healthy fat, and micronutrients.

Makes 4 servings

2 pounds wild-caught tightly closed mussels

2 tablespoons olive oil

1 small yellow onion, diced

2 garlic cloves, minced

1 bunch curly green kale or collard greens, stems removed and sliced into ribbons

Sea salt

1 cup bone broth or vegetable broth

1 bunch fresh parsley, chopped

Broccoli or radish sprouts or other microgreens

Roasted fingerling potatoes, optional

Sourdough bread, optional

Soak the mussels in a large bowl of cold water for 20 minutes. Transfer them to a colander and rinse under cold running water, discarding any damaged or opened mussels. Remove any "beards" (the string hanging from the shell) with a towel.

In a large Dutch oven or stockpot, heat the olive oil over medium heat. Add the onion and gently sauté until translucent, stirring occasionally with a wooden spoon for about 10–15 minutes. Add the garlic, sizzling it in the heat for a minute, then add the kale, briefly cooking until it wilts, about 3 minutes. Season the onion, garlic, and kale mix with salt, keeping in mind that the broth and mussels are salty.

Add the broth and the mussels to the Dutch oven. Cover and cook for 3 to 4 minutes over medium heat until the mussels open and are cooked through on the inside. Discard any unopened mussels. Serve the mussels with the parsley and sprouts sprinkled on top along with roasted fingerling potatoes or sourdough bread, if desired. Savor the broth!

Wakame, Ginger, and Miso Soba Noodles with Avocado

A 2005 study from UC Berkeley found that cisgender women with endometriosis experienced a significant improvement in their symptoms and menstrual irregularities after taking 700 mg of seaweed capsules every day. While we usually eat terrestrial plants, marine plants such as seaweeds offer an abundance of vitamins and minerals and improve estrogen and phytoestrogen metabolism. Wakame and kelp are also especially rich in folate. Seaweed varieties like kelp, dulse, and wakame pair well with soups, mushroom and bone broths, and rice dishes like congee. The following is a soothing broth that you can serve with noodles, additional vegetables, or a soft-boiled egg.

Makes 4 servings

1 package soba noodles (or rice noodles)

5 cups dashi, chicken bone broth, or water

1-inch piece fresh ginger, minced

2 cloves garlic, minced

¼ cup dried wakame

2 cups shiitake mushrooms, stemmed and sliced

2 small bok choy, cleaned and chopped thin

2 tablespoons white miso paste

2 tablespoons shoyu, tamari, or coconut aminos

3 medium carrots, julienned

2 scallions, cut into diagonal slivers

1 cup sugar snap peas, cut into diagonal slivers, optional

Basil leaves

1 avocado, sliced

Lime juice

Seaweed gomasio or sesame seeds

2 soft-boiled eggs, optional

Cook the soba noodles according to the package directions and then rinse them in a colander under cold water. Set aside.

Heat a large Dutch oven over medium heat and add the dashi, ginger, and garlic. Simmer for 5 minutes, then add the wakame, mushrooms, and white parts of the bok choy. Simmer for 8 to 10 minutes.

RECIPE CONTINUES

Spoon the miso paste into a small bowl. Ladle out a few spoonfuls of the broth and add it to the miso, stirring vigorously to combine. Pour the miso broth into the Dutch oven, then stir in the shoyu and the green parts of the bok choy.

Remove the Dutch oven from the heat. Add the cooked soba noodles to individual bowls, ladle broth on top of the noodles, and arrange the carrots, scallions, snap peas, basil leaves, and a few slices of avocado on top. Finish with a squeeze of lime, seaweed gomasio, and soft-boiled eggs, if desired.

Sardine Cakes with Scallions, Parmesan, and Spinach

As much as I love sardines on their own, I understand that many may need a little enticing to get these economical, nutrient-dense, sustainable fish into their mouths. These cakes are a crispy, flavor-packed, sardine delivery system that pretty much everyone can get behind. While I most often make these cakes with sardines, you can make them with almost any canned fish, including salmon, mackerel, and tuna. Sardines are rich in omega-3s—richer in this essential fatty acid than many fish oils. They're also packed with selenium, calcium, phosphorus, and vitamin D, along with other vitamins and minerals.

Makes 12 cakes

One 4½-ounce can wild sardines in extra virgin olive oil

2 eggs

1 teaspoon sea salt

¼ teaspoon ground cumin

¼ teaspoon ground turmeric

⅛ teaspoon cayenne pepper

2 scallions, thinly sliced

1 cup grated parmesan or pecorino

¼ cup parsley, chopped

2 packed cups kale or spinach, finely chopped

1 cup almond flour or oat flour

2 tablespoons olive oil

TO SERVE

1 pound leafy greens such as arugula, mustard greens, or lettuce

1 apple, thinly sliced

Lemon juice

Parmesan, grated

Flaky sea salt

Olive oil

In a large mixing bowl, smash the sardines and the oil they come in together with a fork. Add the eggs and stir to combine. Stir in the salt, spices, scallions, parmesan, parsley, kale, and flour. Heat the olive oil in a large skillet over medium-high heat. Spoon round mounds of the sardine mix into the skillet and fry them until they're golden brown on both sides. Be careful not to overcrowd—I recommend cooking them in two batches.

Serve the sardine cakes on a large bed of leafy greens with the apple slices, lemon juice, more parmesan, flaky sea salt, and a drizzle of olive oil.

Berry, Ginger, and Greens Kefir Smoothie

The word *kefir* comes from the Turkish word *keyif*, which translates into "feeling good." Kefir is the result of the interaction between a liquid such as milk or water and the symbiotic bacteria and yeasts in kefir grains, which are clusters of living microorganisms that consume lactose during the culturing process to create an effervescent, tangy, and drinkable yogurt-like product. Kefir is a probiotic-rich beverage that has antimicrobial, anticancer, antitumor, and immune system–boosting effects. Like other fermented foods, kefir contributes to a healthy gut microbiome, which regulates estrogen metabolism. Look for whole milk kefir, goat milk kefir, or an alternative like coconut milk kefir. Or you can make your own by inoculating whole milk with kefir grains.

Makes 1 serving

2 cups packed spinach

1 cup whole milk kefir or coconut milk kefir

1 cup frozen cherries, blueberries, blackberries, raspberries, or strawberries, or a combination

½-inch piece fresh ginger, grated

1 tablespoon grass-fed beef or plant-based collagen, optional

Ice, optional

Blend all the ingredients together, adding a few handfuls of ice if desired. Enjoy immediately.

Follicular Seed Balls

If you're interested in trying out seed cycling (see page 100), this recipe provides enough balls for the average follicular phase, starting on the first day of your period and ending with the day you ovulate. These energy and nutrient-rich balls are packed with healthy fats and protein from the nuts with just the right amount of sweetness. Pumpkin seeds are a great source of zinc, magnesium, iron, manganese, and copper while flaxseeds are the richest plant-based source of the omega-3 alpha-linolenic acid (ALA), and also contain lignans, fiber, potassium, and protein. Consume one ball a day.

Makes 16 balls

1 cup raw, whole pumpkin seeds

½ cup cashew, almond, or other nut butter

½ cup almond flour

¾ cup ground flaxseeds

¼ cup melted ghee or coconut oil

2 pitted dates, finely chopped

1 teaspoon maple syrup (optional)

¼ teaspoon cinnamon

¼ teaspoon ground ginger

Pinch sea salt

Add all the ingredients to a medium mixing bowl and stir together until thoroughly combined. Using your hands tends to work best.

Using your hands or a cookie scooper, form the mixture into balls slightly larger than a tablespoon and place them onto a baking sheet lined with parchment- or wax-paper. Freeze them until they're solid and then transfer the balls into an airtight container and put them back in the freezer. These will last for a month. When you're ready to enjoy one, allow the seed ball to come to room temperature for a few minutes before eating.

Matcha Cacao and Coconut Butter Cups

Matcha comes from the *Camellia sinensis* plant, which, unlike other green tea, is shade-grown for 20 to 30 days before it is harvested, dried, and ground into a fine powder. The resulting vibrant tea is often referred to as a mood-and-brain food that supports attention, focus, memory, and reaction speed. These benefits are thought to come from antioxidants such as catechins and compounds l-theanine, EGCG (epigallocatechin gallate), and caffeine. These matcha cups made with cacao and coconut butter are a fun and tasty way to enjoy matcha.

Makes 8 matcha cups

1 cup cacao butter

¼ cup coconut butter

4 tablespoons coconut oil

1 tablespoon maple syrup

1 teaspoon matcha powder

Pinch sea salt

Set up a double boiler: In a small saucepan, bring 1–2 inches of water to a simmer, then place a glass bowl over the top so that it sits above—but not touching—the water. Reduce the heat to medium–low. In the glass bowl, combine the cacao butter, coconut butter, coconut oil, maple syrup, matcha powder, and salt. Gently melt the mixture, whisking occasionally until it is completely liquid. Carefully pour the matcha into silicone molds or a muffin tin lined with muffin cups.

Place the silicone molds or muffin tin in the refrigerator (or freezer) and allow the matcha cups to solidify, then enjoy. Store the matcha cups in the refrigerator for up to one week.

Oatstraw Herbal Latte with Milk and Honey

Oatstraw is rich in minerals including iron, calcium, and magnesium. It is well-loved by herbalists for its healing and restorative benefits. This herbal latte is intended to support the energy shift from the follicular to the luteal phase and provides grounded and calm energy. This recipe was developed by the clinical herbalist Mary McCallum.

Makes 1 latte

- 1½ cup water
- 1 tablespoon dried oatstraw powder
- Zest from ½ lemon
- ¼ teaspoon rosehip powder
- 2 tablespoons cream of choice
- 1 teaspoon raw honey

In a small saucepan, heat the water over medium-high heat and whisk in the oatstraw, zest, and rosehip powder until heated through and steaming. Add the cream and honey and whisk again until the latte is blended and frothy. Pour into your favorite mug and enjoy.

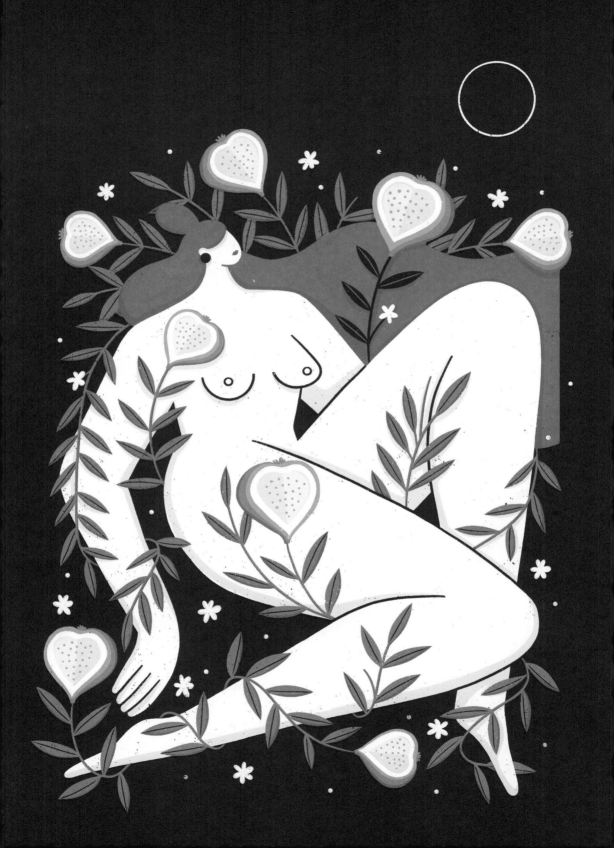

Ovulatory Phase

SUMMER • OPEN + FREE

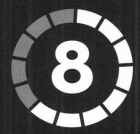

In the late spring and early summer, many trees experience their highest rate of root expansion, along with abundant leaf growth. This growth depends on spring conditions such as having enough water, sunlight, and nutrients. Mature leaves and young stems convert the sun's energy into sugars that sustain and maintain the health of the tree. If the tree is stressed by disease or poor water supply, it uses more of its energy to maintain the current root system and leaves. Whereas, if all the conditions are prime, it can focus on maintenance along with storing nutrients for the seasons ahead while also growing. The summer is an energetic time for the tree; it takes full advantage of the warm weather and sunlight while also maintaining its health and preparing for what's to come in the fall and winter.

Similarly, the ovulatory phase is like a brief summertime, when you might feel especially receptive and vibrant—growing your roots while also feeling a sense of expansion. As much as ovulation is about the present, and specifically the moment when an egg is released from a follicle in one of the ovaries, it's also a moment that is dedicated to the potential for more life in the future.

The short ovulatory phase is a momentous flurry of activity for your body, and it represents the culmination of hormonal activity that urged an egg to burst out of its ovary home and into the fallopian tube. This phase, more than any other, is what the menstrual cycle is all about, and it represents a midway point in our cycle when our energy shifts. According to Traditional Chinese Medicine, ovulation and the associated rise in basal body temperature (BBT) shift our energy from yin to yang, warming the body through the luteal phase. As our estrogen levels rise, the dark and cool energy of yin shifts to the warming, nourishing, rising sun of yang. Yang energy allows our energy to peak, balances the yin energy of menstruation, and is a moment of expansiveness and possibility perfectly encapsulated in this brief body-full moment of summer.

Sexual Motivation and Desire

The hormones involved in ovulation influence our physiology and behavior. Cervical mucus becomes fertile, the endometrium thickens, and breast tissue may feel buoyant or sensitive. At the height of fertility, rising estrogen levels have a slight inhibitory effect on appetite, so we tend to eat fewer calories. As ovulation nears, research finds that naturally cycling people experience increased sexual desire and improved body image; they may feel sexier and masturbate more. A 2018 study that examined 26,000 cisgender straight women's sexual desire and behavior during ovulation found that the women who were naturally cycling experienced an increase in their sexual desire leading up to and during ovulation. This increase in desire was generally aimed at the women's partners, but the paper also found that during peak fertility, cycling women experienced increased sexual interest in their own partners and other men. The study found that the individuals using hormonal contraceptives experienced more of a flat line in their level of sexual desire, which suggests that the hormones that peak just prior to and during ovulation play a role in influencing our interest in sex.

Not only might we feel sexier and desire more sex during peak fertility, but we also tend to feel more positive leading up to and during ovulation. In a small 2017 study in Spain, researchers looked at affect and its relationship to the menstrual cycle. *Affect* is the scientific term used to describe pleasant and unpleasant sensations. Words like engagement, joy, and contentment describe a positive affect while depression, anger, and anxiety describe a negative affect. Our affect contributes to our "orientation to happiness," meaning a person with a generally more positive affect is more likely to look for meaning and pleasure in life and find joy in experiences.

The Spanish study found that naturally cycling cisgender women were more likely to experience increased positive affect and decreased negative affect during ovulation compared to their non-ovulating counterparts who were using hormonal contraceptives. A negative affect tends to make the world feel smaller and narrows thinking, while a positive affect has a broadening effect. This theory—called the "broaden-and-build" theory of positive emotions developed by Dr. Barbara Fredrickson—states that a positive affect encourages us to be more open, engaged, and creative. In this positive emotional state, we feel that we have more options and are able to develop our skills, knowledge, and resources. Ovulating gives us a brief boost—the peak in our hormones and the release of the egg coinciding with a world that feels more expansive and meaningful.

Researchers don't fully understand how sex hormones influence our affect, but the hormones involved in the menstrual cycle appear to induce physical changes in the brain. Right before and during ovulation, naturally cycling individuals self-report increased activity levels, alertness, enthusiasm, and attentiveness. These changes coincide with peak fertility and are often explained as evolutionary adaptations that increase the likelihood of reproduction. The thinking goes that when we're alert, enthusiastic, and positive, we're more likely to get out there and find a sperm-contributing mate so we can reproduce. These changes in female behavior around the time of ovulation build the basis for a theory developed in 1998 called the ovulatory shift hypothesis: sexual motivation increases when the likelihood of conception is highest to improve the chance of conception with a healthy partner with good genes who is also a good co-parent and provider.

Many studies have challenged and rebutted the ovulatory shift hypothesis including a 2019 study from *Evolutionary Psychology*, which found that while people who menstruate experience increased sexual desire and improved body image during ovulation, their mate preference didn't change, meaning when they were ovulating, they didn't suddenly prefer mates with hypermasculine traits (unless they already preferred those mates). The reality is that we're not motivated to have sex *just* to reproduce. Unlike some mammals, like lemurs, who can only mate one or two days out of the year, we (and apparently, dolphins) can have sex year-round for pleasure. Sexual motivation may peak with ovulation, but this increase in sexual desire isn't limited to cisgender straight females seeking to conceive with a cisgender straight male. All of this is to say that when we're feeling more sexual, we're not always hoping to reproduce, and our arousal is not exclusive to any specific gender.

Sex in Context

If sexual motivation can't be simply explained by an innate desire to reproduce, how then can we explain sexuality and how is it affected by our hormones? If we think of sexuality as a complex process that integrates psychological, physiological, and environmental factors, we can see how and why this process is so variable from person to person and throughout the menstrual cycle in the same person. Sexual motivation, or the willingness to engage in sexual behaviors, is a mental state when our interest in sex is heightened and prioritized. It is influenced by psychological and psychosocial factors such as past sexual experiences, our relationship with our partner, self-image, and emotional well-being. Meanwhile, physiological factors in the brain influence both sexual motivation and arousal.

Sexy stimuli, like a steamy lovemaking scene in a movie, activate our visual processing system, which relays information about this sexy scene to certain regions of the brain involved in motivation and reward. Depending on our psychological state and our environment, we might experience an excitatory response or an inhibitory response to this sexual imagery. We can think of an excitatory response as "turned on" and the inhibitory response as "turned off." Some recent studies have looked at how the menstrual cycle influences the brain's response to sexy stimuli. In one study that examined brain activation in response to sexual imagery during ovulation, the researchers found that some regions of the brain experienced a decrease in activation while other regions were activated during this phase. The authors proposed that this change decreased brain processes that inhibit sexual behavior while enhancing the emotional salience of sexual imagery, thus increasing sexual motivation and behavior. In other words, we are both less likely to be turned off and more likely to be turned on when experiencing sexual imagery. Thanks, brain.

Our ovarian hormones do not directly drive our sexual behavior. Rather, they influence certain brain centers, thus influencing sexual behavior and motivation. Estradiol specifically appears to increase our excitatory response to sexual stimuli while simultaneously decreasing inhibitory responses. Sex, and the willingness and motivation to do it, are wrapped up in contexts. Our hormones are part of that context, exerting their influence on certain parts of our brains, but they are not the whole story.

Tracking the Fertile Window

Ovulation is a carefully orchestrated event regulated by our hormones and executed by the ovaries. The actions of the almond-sized ovaries are largely ruled by FSH and LH, which interact with and respond to estrogen and progesterone. Specifically, a surge in LH spurred by a peak in estrogen induces ovulation. LH and progesterone weaken the wall of the ovary, allowing the egg to break free. The LH surge also causes certain cells to form the corpus luteum, a temporary endocrine gland that produces progesterone and estrogen and transitions the body from the ovulatory phase to the luteal phase.

The brief period of time when conception is possible is called the fertile window. From one cycle to the next, the timing of ovulation often varies, so the fertile window also varies. This variability is why it's so important to continually track signs of fertility. The standard clinical guidelines say that the average woman is fertile between day ten and seventeen of her menstrual cycle, assuming that ovulation happens on day fourteen in a twenty-eight-day cycle. But one study found that more than 70 percent of cisgender women are in their fertile window before day ten or after day seventeen, clearly showing this assumption to be outdated and inaccurate. Your fertile window is unique to your cycle and can't be generalized.

If you choose to track your fertile window, you can do so using fertility awareness–based methods (read more about these methods on page 42). Another common method of detecting ovulation is an over-the-counter test kit that measures urinary LH. Multiple studies have shown that LH kits are an accurate, inexpensive, and minimally invasive way to detect ovulation. This method requires testing LH once or twice daily starting on the tenth or eleventh day of the cycle. On average, after a positive LH result, ovulation occurs seventeen to twenty-four hours later. Tracking LH to detect ovulation is still a nuanced art; the LH surge doesn't always indicate ovulation because we don't all surge the same way. Some LH surges are rapid, meaning they happen in one day, while others occur gradually over two to six days. LH surges vary in configuration too. They may be spiking, biphasic, or plateauing, and a small percentage of people (4.3 percent) experience an LH surge without ovulation. Premature LH surges also often fail to trigger ovulation. Like the other fertility awareness methods, urinary LH should not act as a stand-alone method of tracking ovulation.

Recently, ovulation prediction technology has experienced its own surge in innovation. High-tech fertility monitors worn as bracelets, armbands, rings, or inserted vaginally consistently measure core body temperature and use this data to predict the fertile window and the day of ovulation with a high level of accuracy. Some monitors measure electrolyte levels in cervical fluid and saliva while other emerging technologies collect biometric data and use AI to learn and analyze our temperature and sleeping patterns, providing accurate ovulation predictions from month to month. Even though many of these technologies are expensive, this new world of fertility monitoring technology is exciting because it gives people who menstruate another option to track, understand, and manage their fertility.

THE MENSTRUAL CYCLE AFTER A BABY

The time from the birth of a baby until the return of regular menstrual cycles is known as the postpartum transition to fertility. This transition can be challenging to navigate as there is no one-size-fits-all rule for when we become fertile again after pregnancy and childbirth. Indicators of fertility like cervical mucus and basal body temperature can be difficult to interpret during the postpartum transition, and breastfeeding further affects when cycles return. During pregnancy, high levels of progesterone and estrogen inhibit ovulation, which is why pregnant people don't experience a monthly period. After birth, these hormone levels drop dramatically and prolactin (the hormone involved in milk production) and suckling during breastfeeding inhibit the normal release of gonadotropin-releasing hormone (GnRH), LH, and FSH, thus continuing the pause of ovulation. When suckling decreases—usually when other nutrition is introduced to the baby at six months—the ovulation-inhibiting effects of breastfeeding lessen, though the return of fertility is still variable and unpredictable. The duration of breastfeeding, frequency of feeding, pumping milk versus nursing directly from the nipple, and whether we exclusively breastfeed or supplement with formula all affect the postpartum return of fertility.

So the postpartum transition is an excellent time to work with a fertility awareness educator who can help you navigate these shifts and teach you how to track your cycle. Educators certified in the Marquette Method teach a highly effective protocol that identifies the return of fertility and helps you avoid pregnancy with a high rate of success. You might also consider some of the previously mentioned wearable technology that tracks basal body temperature, helping to identify when you first ovulate. This option is especially useful postpartum as you won't have to remember to take your temperature daily while caring for a new baby.

Additionally, your menstrual cycle might change postpartum. For some, it is heavier and more irregular with more cramping, especially the first few cycles. For others, there's less cramping and fewer PMS symptoms. If your vagina is still healing from a vaginal birth, it might be more comfortable to use period underwear or pads, especially if your cycle returns early.

STEPS OF THE POSTPARTUM TRANSITION

1. Immediately after birth, the ovaries are quiet and we do not experience ovulatory cycles or menstruation. Lochia, the normal discharge after birth, lasts up to six weeks. During this time, estrogen and progesterone levels are very low.

2. The ovaries wake up and follicular development resumes. The timing of this varies depending on breastfeeding.

    a. Without breastfeeding, the first menses generally returns between four weeks and three months postpartum.

    b. With breastfeeding, the first menses occurs on average at seven months postpartum and the first ovulation occurs at eight months postpartum. The first menses is usually followed by irregular cycles for three to six months (a long follicular phase and short luteal phase). According to research, by six months postpartum, 20 percent of cisgender breastfeeding women ovulate and 25 percent menstruate. By twelve months, 64 percent have ovulated and 70 percent have menstruated.

3. It is possible for ovulation to occur before the first menses.

    a. Research shows that if you ovulate early during breastfeeding, you're likely to ovulate early with future babies. Likewise, the return of fertility from one baby to the next with similar intensity of breastfeeding happens at about the same time.

4. The luteal phase is often short in length after the first menses (six days or less) and slowly lengthens as the cycle transitions back to normal. Regular cycles resume.

When Ovulation Hurts

Ideally, we experience the ovulatory phase as a high-energy, pain-free, magnetic, and vibrant few days where we feel especially interested in sex and moving our bodies. However, research from the Clue app found that one in three people track pain during ovulation, a phenomenon known as *mittelschmerz* (German for "middle" and "pain"). This pain tends to feel like a dull or sharp cramp in the abdomen on the side where the ovary is releasing the egg. It can last for a few hours or days, may not occur every cycle, and most often occurs on the day prior to or of ovulation. The cause of ovulation pain remains unknown. One theory is that it is a result of inflammatory compounds that spur the release of the egg and other studies show that mittelschmerz coincides with the peak in LH. The medical treatment for ovulation pain, like other cycle-related symptoms, is often NSAIDs or hormonal contraception. Other effective treatments that can help relieve mittelschmerz include taking a hot bath with Epsom salts, using a heating pad on the abdomen, abdominal massage, deep belly breathing, moving your body, and incorporating foods that have an anti-inflammatory effect like ginger and turmeric. If you experience mittelschmerz regularly, it's important to rule out other disorders like abnormal cysts or endometriosis. Tracking ovulation pain—its severity, location, and duration—along with other lifestyle factors such as sleep quality and stress may also give you clues about what makes the pain worse or better. The one benefit of ovulation pain is that it indicates ovulation.

Anovulatory Cycles

What about when ovulation doesn't happen? A cycle without ovulation is called an anovulatory cycle. Occasional anovulatory cycles are normal and common, but consistent anovulatory cycles may indicate an underlying medical condition. Often, anovulatory cycles are longer than ovulatory cycles and you may still experience a period, though it might feel different from ovulatory cycle bleeding both in blood quantity and the PMS symptoms you experience. The most obvious problem with anovulation is infertility for those who want to become pregnant, but ovulation is also an important indicator of overall and hormonal health (note, though, that the purpose of hormonal birth control is to prevent ovulation, and this doesn't make you unhealthy).

The potential causes of an anovulatory cycle are many. Conditions like PCOS, which is the leading cause of infertility and associated with insulin resistance, can disrupt the endocrine system and lead to an anovulatory cycle. Other conditions that are associated with disrupted menstrual cycles include abnormal thyroid or adrenal hormone levels; chronic inflammatory conditions; toxicity from exposure to pesticides, BPA, parabens, and phthalates; too high or too low body weight; and overexercising. The underlying cause of an anovulatory cycle is complex and beyond the scope of this book, so if this is affecting you, you may want to consider working with an OB/GYN or endocrinologist. But there are also some general ways you can improve the likelihood of having an ovulatory cycle.

Movement and Anovulation

A 2017 study from *Sports Medicine* found that people who vigorously exercised for thirty to sixty minutes per day were more likely to experience a cycle with ovulation and that, with or without dietary changes, exercise can lead to the resumption of ovulation in individuals whose previous cycles were anovulatory. In overweight individuals, exercise decreases free androgen levels and lowers insulin, which restores the functioning of the hypothalamus–pituitary–adrenal (HPA) axis and the regulation of ovulation. All of this is to say that movement supports hormonal and overall health.

Importantly, the study also found that individuals who exercise excessively, which varies depending on the person, or who are underweight stress their bodies in a way that may result in HPA dysfunction and a disrupted menstrual cycle. Exercise and the hormones involved in ovulation are tied in other ways too. Rising estrogen levels associated with the preovulatory and ovulatory phase have an impact on our musculoskeletal function and affect the function and structure of our muscles, tendons, and ligaments. Interestingly, estrogen improves the function of bones and muscles, but decreases the stiffness of tendons and ligaments, which can predispose us to ligament injuries. Several studies have found a higher risk of knee ligament injuries during the preovulatory and ovulatory phases compared to the luteal and menstrual phases. But these studies also find that the periodic rise in estrogen before ovulation actually improves how our muscles respond and repair following exercise, leading to stronger tendons, ligaments, and muscles over time. The idea from this research is that while high estrogen levels can increase the risk of injury for a few days of the month, people who are ovulating monthly experience improved musculoskeletal health and performance in the long run.

One way to balance the increased risk of injury during the ovulatory phase is to change how you move. Choosing low-impact activities such as walking and hiking (instead of running, for example) for a few days during your peak estrogen levels and properly warming up your body before exercising may help prevent ligament injuries while benefiting long-term musculoskeletal health.

Self-Care

Turn On

The ovulatory phase is an excellent time to deepen your connection to your sexuality. In her book *Come As You Are*, Emily Nagoski, an expert on sexuality, wrote that "arousal is really two processes: activating the accelerator and deactivating the brakes." Sexual motivation tends to be high during the ovulatory phase, making it a good time to explore your accelerators (what turns you on) and your brakes (what turns you off). If you're ovulating and want to avoid pregnancy, be sure to use a condom or other barrier contraception method if you're having vaginal intercourse with a sperm-contributing partner. But whether or not you're having sex, you can (and should!) also practice self-intimacy, which doesn't necessarily have to be sexual. For example, being aware of your physical sensations, connecting to your body, and showing yourself appreciation by taking care of your spiritual, emotional, and physical needs are ways to practice self-intimacy and love.

Here are a few science-backed ways to improve overall sexual well-being and self-intimacy:

- Practice self-compassion and avoid people or media that make you feel self-critical.

- Treat yourself with kindness and prioritize your needs.

- Set healthy boundaries for yourself with your family, work, and friends.

- Get naked, spend time in front of the mirror, and learn to love, trust, and value your body.

- Masturbate, with or without toys such as vibrators. If you're struggling with orgasm, try Nagoski's therapeutic masturbation recommendations in her book.

Broaden and Build

Positive emotions encourage us to broaden our thinking in ways that are creative, unpredictable, and flexible. They also open our awareness to the world, allowing us to build up our resources so that we're better equipped to solve problems and cope with stress. (Read more about this on page 125.) There are several ways to nurture positive emotions, including spending enjoyable time with family and friends, spending time in nature, practicing gratitude, volunteering our time, supporting others, or giving to causes we believe in. Additionally, acknowledging and expressing negative emotions in a safe space like with a trusted friend, therapist, or through a journaling habit allow us to grow our emotional intelligence as we cultivate a more rational and balanced perspective. Above all, practicing kindness, appreciation, curiosity, authenticity, and sincerity in our daily lives and reinforcing these attributes through practices like mindfulness meditation set up a strong foundation for positive emotions as we move through our lives.

Herbal Flower Soak

This flower-filled bath, developed by the clinical herbalist Mary McCallum, is a celebration of the ovulatory phase meant to honor your creative, confident, and sexy energy. The healing flowers included in this soak reduce muscle tension and are uplifting and sensual. You can put the flowers directly in your tub or use a reusable tea bag to decrease cleanup time.

Makes 1 soak

2 cups Epsom salt

¼ cup rose petals

¼ cup calendula flowers

¼ cup lavender flowers

¼ cup chamomile

3 tablespoons olive oil or almond oil

5–10 drops of essential oil from rose, lavender, sweet orange, helichrysum, or a mix (optional)

In a medium mixing bowl, add the salt and then fold in the rose, calendula, lavender, and chamomile. Stir in the oil and essential oils, if using. Store in a 16-ounce mason jar for later use, use immediately in the bath, or use ½ cup in warm water as a foot soak.

Movement

This short and sweet phase is a perfect opportunity to challenge yourself to tackle a big natural movement goal. For example, go for a five-, ten-, or fifteen-mile hike, try a full-body movement like rock climbing, or go out foraging for mushrooms. Whatever you choose, the peaking hormones of this phase tend to correspond with a peak in energy levels. Keeping in mind the higher risk of ligament injury during this phase (see page 132), we can choose to move in a way that protects our ligaments. The way we move changes with our alignment, and alignment affects where we place loads on our body. When we place excessive loads on our knees because of poor alignment (from wearing shoes with heels, sitting too much, or not moving in diverse ways, for example), we place higher loads on our ligaments, which also puts undue strain on the muscles around the knee. The following movements are helpful for improving alignment along with muscle strength and function. Before you head out for your big ovulatory-phrase adventure, integrate these movements so that you can challenge yourself without injuring your ligaments.

Stretch Your Calves

When our calves are tense, there is often an underlying biomechanical issue that causes shortening of the muscles. Shortened calf muscles are less able to absorb loads when you move and cause tension in the quadricep muscles, which leads to misplaced loads and knee instability and pain. The biomechanist and natural movement expert Katy Bowman recommends stretching your calves by using a half-cylinder foam roller or rolled-up towel. Step onto the roller (or towel) by placing the ball of your foot on the top of the roller and allowing your heel to gently touch the ground. Then, step the opposite foot forward with the stretching leg still on the roller. Keep both legs straight and keep your weight balanced over the stretching leg. You can also slightly bend your knee to deepen the calf stretch. This can be done while you work at a standing desk, while talking on the phone, or before heading out for a walk. Stretch each side for a few minutes and repeat often.

Use Your Butt

Strong muscles in the butt and hips stabilize the sacrum, pelvis, and pelvic floor muscles. The gluteus maximus muscles influence knee movements and coordinate the movements of the pelvis with the spine and lower body. When you use your glutes, you also naturally untuck your pelvis, which helps you stop thrusting your pelvis forward, a common misalignment. A great way to strengthen and protect this area is to engage your glutes and the muscles in your hips and hip flexors as you walk.

Connect to the Earth

A 2012 study published in the *Journal of Environmental and Public Health* found that spending time barefoot on natural surfaces of the earth, also known as earthing or grounding, has surprising health benefits including a reduction in inflammation and pain, decreased blood viscosity, chronic stress reduction, regulation of the nervous system, improved sleep, and other body-wide benefits. This paper and others propose that bodily connection (we don't only have to use our feet) to the Earth's surface electrons has a stabilizing effect on our physiology and increases well-being. Supported by a surprising amount of research, earthing is easy and accessible; the authors of the study recommend thirty- to forty-minute daily barefoot sessions on naturally conductive surfaces such as grass, gravel, soil, stone, and sand to reap the benefits.

Move Mindfully

Most knee ligament injuries are sports-related and occur from sharp movements such as pivoting. Pay attention to where you're stepping and how your body is moving as a whole so that you can avoid placing unnecessary strain on your knees. Additionally, choose a movement goal that is appropriate for you. For example, if you regularly hike ten miles, challenge yourself to hike fifteen or twenty miles, but if the farthest you've hiked is two miles, perhaps challenge yourself to hike four miles. Start slow and build a balanced, stable, strong, and flexible body. Your ligaments will thank you.

OVULATORY PHASE
Recipes

Purple Sauerkraut

Making your own sauerkraut is one of the simplest, most economical ways to get more beneficial fermented foods into your life. I tend to make a batch once a month and eat the kraut with most of my meals. Fermented foods improve the health of the gut microbiome, which is one of the key regulators of circulating estrogens. The purple cabbage is particularly pretty, but you can use any color of cabbage you wish.

Makes around 5 cups of sauerkraut

1 large or 2 small purple cabbages (about 5 pounds)

2½ tablespoons sea salt (1 tablespoon salt for every 2 pounds of cabbage)

Remove any damaged, browned, or wilted-looking outer leaves and cut each cabbage in half, cutting out the nub at its base, then cut into quarters. Slice the quarters into thin ribbons. Place the cabbage in a large mixing bowl and toss it with the sea salt. Allow the mix to sit for thirty minutes and then give the cabbage a nice, strong massage for a few minutes.

Place the cabbage in a fermentation vessel (a fermentation crock or mason jars) and using your fist, press the cabbage down into the vessel. The goal is to get the liquid that naturally comes out of the cabbage when you massage it with salt to completely cover the cabbage. If you need to, you can add a little salt water. Weight the cabbage with fermentation weights or a baggy full of water and cover with a lid. Allow the kraut to ferment in a cool dark place out of direct sunlight.

After 5 days, the sauerkraut is ready to eat, but you can also let it sit for 2 to 3 weeks depending on your taste preferences. The longer the kraut ferments, the more pungent and funky it tastes, which some people prefer. Fermentation speed also depends on the ambient temperature—kraut stored in warmer temperatures will ferment faster than colder temps. I usually ferment mine for 5 days in the summer and a week or so in the winter. Store extra kraut in the refrigerator and use it within 3 months.

Wild Salmon and Salmon Roe Temaki (Hand Rolls)

Wild salmon and salmon roe are rich sources of omega-3 fatty acids and DHA. Salmon roe is prized by many cultures as an essential and sacred fertility food because of the belief that roe contains the nutrition needed for proper development. It is exceptionally high in omega-3s, vitamin D, vitamin B_{12}, choline, selenium, iron, magnesium, and other trace minerals. Research shows that fish roe may be neuroprotective and beneficial to people with depression, inflammation, autoimmune diseases such as rheumatoid arthritis, and cardiovascular disease.

Makes 6 salmon rolls

2 tablespoons olive oil

12 ounces wild fresh salmon

Sea salt and fresh ground black pepper

2 teaspoons shoyu, tamari, or coconut aminos, plus extra for serving

Toasted nori sheets, cut in half

1 avocado, thinly sliced

Sprouts (preferably radish or broccoli)

Quick Pickled Radishes and Carrots (recipe follows)

Little gem or other sturdy lettuce leaves

Kimchi

Wild salmon roe

Wasabi dipping sauce (optional)

Heat the oil in a skillet over medium-high heat. Season the salmon on both sides with salt and pepper. Place the salmon in the skillet skin side down then drizzle with the shoyu. Cover and cook until the middle is cooked through but still tender and flaky (5 to 8 minutes). Place the salmon on a large plate and using a fork, flake the salmon into long pieces. Don't discard the skin! It's the tastiest part.

For easy rolling, set out the ingredients in this order: nori, lettuce, avocado slices, sprouts, quick pickled veggies, kimchi, cooked salmon, and roe. Place the nori in your hand, shiny side down. Put the lettuce leaf on the left side of the nori and cover it with avocado, sprouts, pickled veggies, kimchi, cooked salmon, and roe. Roll the bottom left corner to the middle of the top-right edge to create a cone shape, and enjoy on its own or with some shoyu and wasabi dipping sauce.

Quick Pickled Radishes and Carrots

Brining vegetables in salt, vinegar, water (and often sugar and spices) is a common way to preserve and add complex flavor. Quick pickling doesn't require canning. Therefore, the pickles must be stored in the refrigerator and used within a month. You can pickle just about any vegetable such as green beans, red onion, asparagus, and of course, cucumbers. Make these at least two hours before use so the flavors have time to develop.

Makes 32 ounces

1 bunch radishes, thinly sliced (use a sharp knife or mandoline)

5 medium carrots, julienned

1 teaspoon salt

1 teaspoon coconut palm sugar (optional)

½ teaspoon red pepper flakes (optional)

¾ cup apple cider vinegar

¾ cup boiling water

Pack the radishes and carrots into a 32-ounce mason jar. Sprinkle the salt over the veggies along with the sugar and red pepper flakes, if using. Pour the vinegar on top, then pour in the boiling water. Allow to cool uncovered to room temperature, then add the lid and shake slightly to incorporate everything. Refrigerate and use after two hours.

Store the pickled veggies in the refrigerator until ready to serve. They will keep for up to a month.

Stir-Fried Forbidden Rice with Mustard Greens, Cabbage, Broccoli Sprouts, and Egg

Cruciferous vegetables such as mustard greens, cabbage, broccoli, brussels sprouts, cauliflower, kale, and collard greens contain compounds that promote the efficient metabolism of estrogen into "good" metabolites that benefit our overall health instead of "bad" metabolites that can contribute to heavy periods, weight gain, and mood disorders. Perfect for those days when you want something quick, nutritious, and almost addictively tasty, this recipe is easy to make and also one of my favorite lunches to bring to work or eat as leftovers.

Makes 4 servings

3 tablespoons shoyu, tamari, or coconut aminos

1-inch piece ginger, grated

1 garlic clove, grated

4 eggs

½ teaspoon salt

6 tablespoons olive oil or grapeseed oil, divided

½ head napa cabbage, quartered and roughly chopped

1 bunch mustard greens, stems removed and chopped

1 bunch scallions, cut into 1-inch pieces

2 cups cooked forbidden rice (1 cup uncooked rice)

1 tablespoon sesame oil

1 tablespoon rice vinegar

TO SERVE, OPTIONAL

Broccoli sprouts

Cilantro, roughly chopped

Avocado slices

Lemon or lime juice

Kimchi

In a small bowl, mix together the shoyu, ginger, and garlic. In another small bowl, whisk the eggs together with the salt.

Heat 2 tablespoons of grapeseed oil in a large cast iron skillet over medium-high. Add the cabbage, cover, and cook for 3 to 4 minutes, then uncover and add the mustard greens and scallions. Cook until the vegetables are charred, about 10 minutes, stirring occasionally.

RECIPE CONTINUES

Transfer the veggies to a medium mixing bowl. Add 2 tablespoons of grapeseed oil to the same skillet and then add the rice. Use the back of a wooden spoon to spread the rice out and gently press it into the skillet, then cook it over high heat until nicely crisped.

While the rice crisps, heat 2 tablespoons of grapeseed oil in another small skillet. Pour in the eggs and stir to scramble until they are just barely set, then remove from the heat.

Add the eggs and shoyu mixture to the rice, tossing well to combine, and then allow the mixture to cook over medium-high heat undisturbed for 4 to 5 minutes. Add the veggies to the skillet and stir to combine. Then remove the skillet from heat and add the sesame oil and rice vinegar, tossing again to combine.

Serve with broccoli sprouts, cilantro, avocado, a squeeze of lemon or lime juice, and kimchi, if desired.

Crispy Pastured Pork Larb with Little Gem Lettuce and Herbs

Larb is a popular dish in Laos and Thailand that marries richly flavorful ground meat with crunchy, colorful vegetables. What I love most about this meal is the abundance of fresh herbs and eating it in the traditional way—with my hands. Herbs contain high levels of antioxidants, they are anti-inflammatory, and the ones in this recipe—basil, cilantro, and mint—protect us against pathogenic bacteria, fungi, and viruses. This is a perfect, light, yet nutrient-dense meal to enjoy during the ovulatory phase.

Makes 6 servings

2 tablespoons ghee or olive oil

2 shallots, peeled and thinly sliced

3 cloves garlic, thinly sliced

1-inch piece fresh ginger, minced

1 Thai red chili

1 pound ground pastured pork (grass-fed ground beef or crumbled tempeh work too)

Sea salt and fresh ground black pepper

1 tablespoon fish sauce (I like Red Boat.)

2 tablespoons shoyu, tamari, or coconut aminos

¼ cup lime or lemon juice

½ cup each fresh basil, cilantro, and mint, plus more for serving

3 scallions, thinly sliced

TO SERVE

Little gem (or other sturdy lettuce) leaves, washed and dried

Lacto-Fermented Ginger and Turmeric Carrots (see page 110) and/or Purple Sauerkraut (see page 138)

Avocado slices

Heat the ghee in a large cast iron skillet over medium-high heat. Add the shallots and cook until they start to sweat, then add the garlic, ginger, and chili and cook for 1 minute.

RECIPE CONTINUES

Add the pork. Season with salt and pepper. Break up the meat with a spatula and press it into the cast iron so that it thoroughly browns. Flip, season, and brown the meat on the other side.

Add the fish sauce and shoyu and cook for another minute. Remove from the heat and stir in the lime juice, fresh herbs, and scallions.

To serve, set up the lettuce leaves, pork mixture, extra herbs, fermented veggies, and avocado slices all in separate bowls. Everyone can make their own larb lettuce wraps by spooning the pork mixture into the lettuce leaves and adding the toppings.

Grass-Fed Beef Liver with Sauteed Apples and Parsley

Allow me for a moment to wax rhapsodic about the superfood that is grass-fed beef liver. Liver: you were once cherished and revered as a treasured food source, recognized for your almost unbelievable nutrient density. You are loaded with the good stuff we need such as vitamin B_{12}, vitamin A, riboflavin, folate, iron, copper, and choline, and yet so many people don't even know about you. But I am on your team, liver. Slowly but surely, intrepid liver lovers like myself are working to bring you back into our collective cultural psyche and kitchens and show you off as a powerful, essential fertility food that, if treated with attention and care, tastes damn good too.

Makes 1 serving

2 tablespoons ghee, butter, or olive oil, plus more as needed

1 apple, cut in half, cored, and thinly sliced

½ cup coarsely chopped parsley

3 ounces grass-fed beef liver, sliced very thin with a sharp knife (this works best if frozen)

Sea salt and fresh ground black pepper

TO SERVE

Leafy greens such as arugula or baby kale

Olive oil

Lemon juice

Sea salt

Heat the ghee in a cast iron skillet over medium heat. Add the apple slices and cook until softened and slightly browned on both sides. Increase the heat to medium-high and add the parsley. Quickly stir the parsley and apple together, then move them to one side of the pan. Add more ghee if needed, then place the liver slices in the skillet, season with salt and pepper, and quickly sear on both sides until browned.

Toss the liver, apples, and parsley together and serve on a bed of leafy greens topped with olive oil, a squeeze of lemon, and sea salt.

Roasted Cod and Asparagus with Herb Butter

If there is a dish that captures the energy of summer, this is it. Low-key but delicious and easy to make, this is what I make after a long day in the sun when I want to eat outside as the sun goes down and the warmth of the summer lingers in the air. Wild-caught cod is a rich source of protein, B vitamins, omega-3 fatty acids, and it is a flavorful, flaky, tender fish. Asparagus is a good source of prebiotics, folate, vitamins A, C, and K, and minerals iron and potassium. Choose in-season, freshly harvested asparagus if possible; it is usually available in the spring and early summer.

Makes 4 servings

1 bunch (about 1 pound) asparagus

1 pound wild cod

Sea salt

Olive oil

Pepper

2 tablespoons Herb Butter (recipe follows), plus more to serve

Lemon juice, to serve

Preheat the oven to 425°F. Snap the woody ends off the asparagus and salt the cod on both sides with a teaspoon of sea salt. Arrange the cod skin side down and asparagus on a baking sheet lined with parchment paper. Drizzle everything with olive oil, season with more salt and pepper, and add the herb butter on top of the cod. Roast until the asparagus spears are easily pierced with a fork and the cod is flaky, but not overcooked, 15–25 minutes depending on the thickness of the fish and the asparagus. Serve with more herb butter and lemon juice.

Herb Butter

Makes about ¾ cups

1 bunch parsley, leaves only

1 clove garlic, minced

2 scallions, roughly chopped

1 lemon, zest and juice

½ teaspoon red pepper flakes (optional)

½ teaspoon sea salt

1 stick (½ cup) room temperature unsalted butter

Put the parsley, garlic, scallions, lemon zest and juice, red pepper flakes (if using), salt, and a grind of pepper in a food processor and pulse until the herbs are finely chopped. Add the butter and pulse until the mixture is smooth and creamy. You can store the herb butter in a container or roll it into a log in some parchment paper and refrigerate it until it solidifies. Use any extra herb butter on fresh, seasonal vegetables, steak, or other fish. Keep refrigerated and use within one week.

Oysters with Pomegranate Vinaigrette

Oysters taste like the ocean—briny, fresh, sweet, and salty. They are full of zinc, selenium, iron, vitamin B_{12}, and vitamin D. When the oysters are fresh, my favorite way to eat these bivalves is raw due to their texture, flavor, and appearance. But I more often eat canned oysters and use them in stews, pastas, or spooned onto sourdough bread or salads the same way you might eat tinned fish. However, for special occasions, this recipe for fresh oysters is especially festive with red pomegranate and green cilantro, though the oysters are equally good with a simple squeeze of lemon.

Makes 24 oysters, or enough for two oyster lovers

2 dozen oysters (see note)

Crushed ice

Pomegranate Vinaigrette (recipe follows)

Cilantro

NOTE: Be sure to get high-quality, super fresh, raw, shucked oysters (you can also shuck them at home). Keep the oysters very cold until you're ready to eat them and toss any that are open or have broken shells.

Serve the raw oysters on a bed of crushed ice with the pomegranate vinaigrette and small leaves of cilantro on top of the oysters.

Pomegranate Vinaigrette

1 tablespoon pomegranate molasses or raw honey

2 tablespoons white wine vinegar or champagne vinegar

2 tablespoons extra virgin olive oil

Seeds from 1 pomegranate

1 small shallot, finely chopped

Fresh ground black pepper

In a small bowl, combine the pomegranate molasses, vinegar, and oil and then stir in the pomegranate seeds and shallot. Season with pepper to taste. Use within one week.

Plentiful Greens Oat Flour Pancakes

These pancakes are a staple in my home because they are quick to make, easily doubled, and crowd-pleasing with their vibrant green color. They are especially tasty with whipped ricotta and seasonal fruit. Spinach and eggs yolks are rich in folate, a key nutrient for fertility health. If you want to up the folate amount even more, you could serve these pancakes with sunflower seed butter, which you can find at most grocery stores.

Makes 4 pancakes

2 packed cups spinach

1½ cups oat flour

1 cup whole milk or nondairy milk of choice

2 eggs

2 tablespoons chia seeds

1 teaspoon baking powder

1 teaspoon apple cider vinegar

¼ teaspoon salt

Butter or ghee

OPTIONAL
TOPPINGS TO SERVE

Berries or other seasonal fruit

Full-fat Greek yogurt or whipped ricotta

Maple syrup

Put all the ingredients except the butter in a blender and blend until smooth.
Heat a tablespoon of butter in a cast iron skillet over medium heat. Spoon ½ cup of batter into the heated pan and fry until golden on both sides. Add more butter as needed for each pancake.
Serve the pancakes hot with the toppings of your choice.

Sprouted Grain-Free Granola with Cacao Nibs

Almost every morning, I eat two breakfasts. First, I go savory: eggs with vegetables and pastured bacon. A few hours later, I go sweet: fresh fruit with plain, whole fat yogurt, and granola. This is my favorite granola for my second breakfast. Not too sweet, but still a treat, it pairs perfectly with yogurt and all kinds of fruits. Nuts and seeds are packed with excellent nutrients such as protein and fiber. Cacao nibs are rich in magnesium. The chia and flaxseeds add omega-3s. Serving this granola with your favorite (dairy or nondairy) plain full-fat yogurt adds a dose of gut-health-promoting probiotics.

Makes 5 cups

1½ cups organic nuts (almonds, cashews, pecans, walnuts, or a mix)

½ cup pumpkin seeds

½ cup raw cacao nibs

1½ cup unsweetened shredded coconut

2 tablespoons chia seeds

2 tablespoons flaxseeds

¼ cup butter

¼ cup olive oil

¼ cup maple syrup or raw honey

½ teaspoon salt

¼ cup currants or dried cherries

TO SERVE, OPTIONAL

Seasonal fruit

Plain full-fat yogurt

Cinnamon

Preheat the oven to 275°F.

In a large mixing bowl, combine the nuts, pumpkin seeds, cacao nibs, shredded coconut, chia seeds, and flax seeds.

In a small saucepan, melt the butter over low heat and then stir in the olive oil, maple syrup, and salt. Pour the melted butter mixture over the nut mixture and stir to evenly coat. Spread the granola in an even layer on a parchment-lined or unlined baking sheet and bake for 1½–2 hours, stirring every 30 minutes.

Remove the granola from the oven and stir in the currants. Serve with the toppings of your choice. Store the granola in an airtight container. Use within one week if stored at room temperature and within one month if frozen.

Hawthorn Rose Syrup

Rose is considered by many herbalists to support energy and creativity, while hawthorn is a traditional medicine for the heart—both the physiological functioning of the organ itself and as energy medicine. Together, these herbs are believed to increase our receptivity to give and receive love and our healing capabilities and courage in the face of heartbreak. I like to add a tablespoon of this syrup to sparkling water or a few spoonfuls to my yogurt, fruit, and granola snack from the previous recipe. Or pour a heaping spoonful over porridge or vanilla ice cream. The floral, sweet syrup elevates simple treats into an elegant dessert. This recipe was developed by the clinical herbalist Mary McCallum.

Makes 16 ounces

2 cups water

1 ounce dried hawthorn berries

½ ounce dried pink rosebuds or rose petals

1 cup raw honey

In a medium saucepan, bring the water to a simmer and then add the hawthorn berries and rosebuds. Simmer over low heat for 15 minutes.

Using a fine mesh sieve, strain and discard the herbs. Pour the infused water back into the saucepan, stir in the honey, and bring to a low simmer for 10 minutes. Turn off the heat, cover the saucepan, and let the infused honey sit for 15 to 20 minutes.

Label a 16-ounce mason jar with the date and name of the syrup, tightly screw on the lid, and store it in the refrigerator. Use within a month of making.

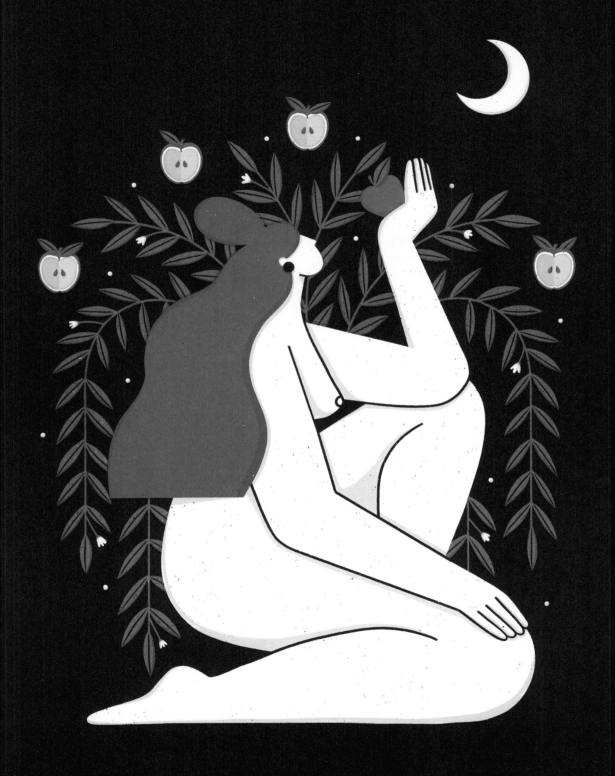

Luteal Phase

FALL • FOCUSED ATTENTION + SENSITIVITY

During the height of the growing season in the summer, trees create chlorophyll—the green pigment that facilitates photosynthesis—at the same rate as they use it so their leaves stay bright green. As the days grow shorter, the production of chlorophyll slows and eventually stops. With decreasing levels of chlorophyll, we can see oranges, yellows, and browns from carotenoids and other pigments present in the leaves. Finally, the leaves—designed to eventually fall from what is called an abscission layer where the leaf stem meets the tree—stop receiving water and nutrients and detach, their life cycle complete for the season.

Fall is a season of transition that includes both late summer and the first signs of winter. Similarly, the luteal phase is composed of the early luteal phase following ovulation when levels of estrogen and progesterone gradually increase and a late luteal phase when the levels of these hormones start to fall and the body prepares for its seasonal shedding. Because this phase is two-in-one, it is one of the more complex phases, and you may experience totally different sensations depending on which day of the luteal phase you're at.

The luteal phase, which lasts from the day of ovulation until the start of the next period, is a season of paying attention to your body, both physically and emotionally. It is a time to be gentle with yourself and mindful of your energy. On average, the luteal phase is twelve to sixteen days long, and after the flurry of spring and summer, fall is marked by a feeling of slowing down and acknowledging change. Common experiences of the luteal phase include a sense of inner quiet, a desire to nest and rest, and an increased sense of clarity and focus. For some, a burst of energy comes in the days leading up to the menstrual phase; for others, PMS symptoms may show up, usually the week before bleeding begins.

Premenstrual Syndrome (PMS)

Emerging research finds that progesterone and estrogen have an impact on our brain connectivity in a way that deeply affects our emotional life. The change in brain connectivity during the late luteal phase appears to be linked to changes in our emotional state about a week before menstruation. For example, some studies show that when cisgender female participants received sex hormones that mimicked the menstrual cycle, they reported an increase in negative mood and enhanced stress response, they remembered negative information better, and some experienced greater emotional distress in the days before they started their period. Negative moods are not universally experienced in the days before menstruation, but for some people, the week leading up to their periods is a time of increased vulnerability to emotional distress.

Studies also show that the prevalence of PMS is higher among Western women as compared to those in other cultures and that PMS symptoms vary across cultures and between ethnic groups. For example, cisgender

American women are more likely to experience negative mood symptoms whereas Chinese women report higher sensitivity to cold. Another study found that African American women were less likely than white women to experience anxiety, crying, and cramps, but more likely to experience headache, fatigue, weight gain, and swelling. More research is needed about PMS across diverse ethnic and cultural groups, but what scientists find is that most people who menstruate experience PMS symptoms, but the language they use to describe the symptoms and the type and severity of symptoms differ.

Though the way we experience PMS is influenced by our culture, it is important to make the distinction that the condition itself isn't made up. It is very real, as those who experience PMS symptoms can attest. Part of the reason we experience PMS differently from culture to culture is because attitudes about menstruation are culturally adopted from how the media and/or our parents talk (or don't talk) about menstruation. The historical rhetoric surrounding the menstrual cycle has taught us to attach negative feelings to the late luteal phase and menstruation. This negativity has complex roots, but is reinforced by some religions and, although this is slowly starting to change, many companies have financially benefited from maintaining period stigma. For example, period products are sold as "sanitary" options for "feminine hygiene," implying that menstruating is unsanitary, unhygienic, and feminine, which excludes people who menstruate who don't identify as women. Washes, creams, and wipes are marketed to "cleanse" and "freshen" the vulva and vagina of "feminine odors," promoting body shame and the false and damaging idea that the vagina needs purifying, deodorizing, and cleaning (it doesn't).

Research shows that our attitudes toward menstruation are influenced by how it is described (as a positive, negative, or neutral event). A study examining attitudes toward menstruation found that as compared to Indian women, who reported that they mostly received positive or neutral information about menstruation, American women reported receiving negative information about menstruation from multiple sources including films, TV shows, cartoons, advertisements, and other popular media. The way we learn to think about our bodies and menstruation matters because, as the authors of this study wrote, "Women's status in a particular society and that society's cultural beliefs about women's bodies shape women's attitudes toward and experiences with their menstrual cycles."

A 2004 paper from *Social Theory & Health* examined the premenstrual experience of seventy cisgender women and argued that the tendency for women to blame their bodies for depressive or angry feelings is rooted in self-policing. Self-policing maintains what the French philosopher Michel

Foucault described as the "pathologization of difference" and is tied to idealized Western notions of femininity that position women as emotional nurturers who sacrifice themselves to take care of their children and their husbands. PMS symptoms juxtapose the accepted mode of femininity and are associated with feelings of guilt, shame, and a lack of control that we blame on our bodies. The authors wrote that learning about and identifying self-policing practices allow people who menstruate to develop an empowering ethic of self-care during the premenstrual phase that may prevent or reduce premenstrual distress.

We can challenge the learned habit of self-policing when we reject unrealistic ideals of what society tells us femininity means and replace blaming our bodies for our symptoms with taking care of our bodies. In one study where women reported higher levels of self-care, received more support, and reevaluated roles and responsibilities in the home, they experienced a significant decrease in premenstrual symptoms and PMS was no longer conceptualized as a problem caused by unruly hormones.

Treating PMS Symptoms

PMS is usually described as a psychological or biological problem. This reductionist explanation leaves out the impact of self-policing and societal constructs that lead us to disregard our own needs for space and self-care, which in turn can exacerbate any symptoms we may be experiencing. It's important to note that there are over 150 symptoms linked to PMS, meaning the variability in experience is huge from person to person. It is helpful to keep track of our personal experience through charting or by recording symptoms in a period tracker app (like Clue, Flo, or Ovia). To qualify as a PMS symptom, the symptom must meet a few criteria: it must recur for at least two previous menstrual cycles during the luteal phase (not before ovulation) and disappear completely after menstruation. If the symptoms don't meet these criteria, it is important to rule out other underlying medical conditions. Additionally, if the PMS symptoms are severe—whether that means severe pain, disturbances in mood, or other symptoms that reduce your quality of life—visit a qualified medical provider.

There are several evidence-based ways to reduce and treat PMS symptoms including non-pharmacologic therapies like cognitive behavioral therapy (CBT) and stress and relaxation techniques. Improved overall health via eating habits, sleep hygiene, and consistent movement practices have also been shown to help reduce PMS symptoms. Other evidence-based therapies that have been shown to help with mild to moderate PMS include calcium supplementation (500–1,200 mg/day), eliminating or reducing alcohol intake, chasteberry (*Vitex agnus castus*) supplements, and vitamin B₆. One study showed that a magnesium supplement combined with vitamin B₆ (250 mg magnesium plus 40 mg B₆ for two months) significantly reduced PMS symptoms such as depression, anxiety, bloating, and lower back pain. In the case of PMS symptoms that are unresponsive to lifestyle changes, medical providers most often prescribe antidepressants and hormonal contraceptives.

Here, it is crucial to point out that premenstrual dysphoric disorder (PMDD), which is marked by severe depressive episodes during the luteal phase, is not just bad PMS. If you are experiencing suicidal thoughts and severe depression and anxiety, seeking professional medical treatment is essential.

THE LIFE AND DEATH OF CORPUS LUTEUM

We can think of the corpus luteum, a temporary endocrine organ, as the director of the uterus during the luteal phase. The hormones it secretes tell the uterus how to adequately prepare its environment for potential implantation, and then it signals when it's time to shed the inner lining. The fate of the corpus luteum is determined by the presence or absence of a fertilized egg. Let's do a little recap: During the preovulatory phase, estrogen thickens the endometrium, and during the luteal phase, progesterone stops the endometrium from continuing to thicken and increases blood supply so that it's ready for possible implantation by a fertilized egg. If fertilization occurs, hCG keeps the corpus luteum around, and it continues to secrete progesterone to maintain the lining of the uterus and the growing embryo. Eventually, the corpus luteum degenerates around week twelve of gestation, when the placenta takes over.

In the absence of a fertilized egg, the corpus luteum retires sooner. After ovulation, it predominately secretes progesterone and estrogen. Progesterone levels peak mid-luteal phase and then start to decrease as the corpus luteum breaks down, around nine or ten days after ovulation.

"Estrogen Dominance" and PCOS

One condition we tend to hear a lot about during the luteal phase is what is commonly referred to as "estrogen dominance," or when a person has high estrogen levels in relation to progesterone or an excess amount of estrogen with low levels of progesterone. Like "hormone balance," "estrogen dominance" isn't an official medical diagnosis; it is used conversationally and in alternative medicine to describe a constellation of symptoms that may occur throughout the cycle, but especially during the luteal phase, such as fatigue, weight gain around the hips, mood changes, and poor sleep. Like Lara Briden, a naturopathic doctor and menstrual cycle expert, I prefer not to use the term "estrogen dominance" because it's vague and doesn't give us information about whether we're ovulating each month, which is the key to progesterone production because ovulation results in the creation of the corpus luteum, which secretes progesterone. Instead, she proposes the more precise terminology of *anovulation*—which can result in low progesterone—*progesterone deficiency*, or *estrogen excess*. As we saw in the last chapter, several conditions may result in anovulation (see page 131), but let's take a closer look at polycystic ovary syndrome (PCOS).

PCOS is a chronic inflammatory condition and one of the most common hormonal disorders in reproductive-age cisgender women. It's characterized by irregular and anovulatory periods, high androgen hormone levels resulting in symptoms like acne and excess facial and body hair (what is called hirsutism), and polycystic ovaries (which are seen on an ultrasound). If you experience at least two of these symptoms, your medical provider will test your testosterone levels, glucose tolerance, cholesterol, and triglycerides. The primary treatment for PCOS is improving overall health via diet and exercise, and/or progesterone therapy, birth control pills, or other medications. Additionally, a 2020 review in *Frontiers in Pharmacology* found that some herbal medicines help ovulation to resume and regulate the menstrual cycle in people with PCOS by decreasing androgens, increasing progesterone, and improving insulin and fat metabolism. This review included many different herbs, both individual extracts and formulations, but a few with beneficial effects included aloe vera gel, Bai zhu (often used in Traditional Chinese Medicine), chamomile, flaxseed, fennel seeds, ginger, and Korean red ginseng. If you're interested in trying herbal therapies for PCOS, it's important to work with a medical provider who understands both PCOS and herbal therapies.

Progesterone is the star hormone of the luteal phase. When progesterone is low, or deficient, our body gives us signs. We may have a short luteal phase (less than eleven days), irregular bleeding or spotting, and a lower basal body temperature (progesterone increases body temperature). Ruling out thyroid disease and underlying inflammatory conditions like PCOS are important first steps to take if you notice signs of estrogen excess or progesterone deficiency during this phase. You can also have your progesterone levels tested mid-luteal phase, around a week before you menstruate, which will tell you if you ovulated that cycle (normal levels vary from person to person and from cycle to cycle, but the normal range for mid-luteal phase progesterone is 2–25 ng/mL). Hormonal health is directly tied to overall health. So, however you experience the luteal phase, taking care of yourself by getting enough sleep, eating well, moving your body, and managing stress helps support progesterone production and a healthy luteal phase.

CULTIVATING HEALTHY SLEEP

Bacteria, fish, reptiles, amphibians, fungi, plants, and mammals such as humans evolved circadian clocks that measure the passage of time on a twenty-four-hour scale. The evolutionary reason for circadian clocks is simple: they are essential for survival under natural conditions and give organisms who have them, like us, an adaptive advantage by syncing our behavior and physiology to our environment. Circadian rhythms include a number of biological rhythms in the human body that cycle on a twenty-four-hour circadian clock. These rhythms are set by specific cells that are regulated by the suprachiasmatic nucleus (SCN)—a group of neurons in the brain. Our circadian rhythm regulates behavioral and physiological changes each day, ranging from eating habits and mood to hormone release and sleep.

We can think of natural conditions as living like our hunter-gatherer ancestors did—that is, without modern conveniences like temperature-regulated homes and artificial light from electricity and devices. Before we could turn on a light when the sun went down or look at our phone in bed, our circadian rhythms didn't get so easily disrupted. Our built environment has changed our relationship to natural light and dark cycles, which throws off our circadian rhythm. The menstrual cycle is a longer biological rhythm, called an infradian rhythm, and it also affects our circadian rhythm, meaning that our sleep changes throughout the menstrual cycle. During the luteal and menstrual phases, the rhythm of melatonin and cortisol release may be blunted, and sleep quality (though subjective) is the lowest during the menstrual phase. Poor sleep quality and a disrupted circadian rhythm are associated with menstrual disorders including PMS, painful menstrual cramping, and irregular menstrual cycles. In the days leading up to and during menstruation, sleep struggles are common, so we must pay close attention to our habits and do our best to realign our circadian clocks to give ourselves the best chance at a quality night's sleep.

Get in Sync with Your Sleep

- **Practice good sleep hygiene.** This is different for everyone, but the basic idea is to create as natural an environment as possible for your circadian rhythm to do its work. Avoid caffeine intake, especially after noon. Limit exposure to blue light for two to three hours before bed and use candles, salt lamps, amber-spectrum light sources, or amber glasses at night so you don't disrupt your melatonin production. Spend time before bed doing relaxing practices such as reading (not on a device), writing, meditating, taking a bath, having sex, etc. Sleep in a cool, completely dark room. Go to bed and wake up at the same time each day and get at least seven hours of sleep.

- **Get light exposure.** Go outside for a walk, ideally between 8 a.m. and 10 a.m., for at least fifteen minutes. This exposure to natural light, preferably sunlight, resets your cortisol rhythm and helps improve mood and energy all day. Use light-box therapy if getting outside in the morning isn't possible.

- **Move your body.** Regularly moving your body helps restore dysregulated circadian rhythms. Sleep and exercise have a bidirectional relationship, meaning poor sleep is associated with low levels of physical activity while more sleep allows for higher levels of physical activity. (See page 170 for more information about supportive movement practices for this phase.)

- **Eat healthy food.** Inflammation and elevated blood glucose from eating excess sugar and processed foods can cause cortisol disturbances (see more about cortisol on page 203). Instead, consider anti-inflammatory foods like vegetables and whole, nutrient-dense foods to support healthy cortisol secretion and rhythms. Avoid or limit alcohol intake before bed as it can disrupt sleep cycles.

The Brain during the Luteal Phase

There is a harmony to the menstrual cycle that is supported by progesterone and estrogen and the complex interplay between these hormones and certain neurotransmitters and neurosteroids. First, a few helpful definitions, and then we'll get into the brain. Neurotransmitters are chemicals that allow brain cells to talk to each other and the rest of the body. Serotonin, dopamine, GABA, and glutamate are major neurotransmitters that interact with our sex hormones. Neurosteroids come from circulating steroid hormones in the brain, and the main one we'll look at in this section is allopregnanolone (ALLO). Progesterone is the precursor steroid for ALLO, which has antianxiety, anti-stress, anticonvulsant, sedative, and neuroprotective benefits.

ALLO levels rise along with progesterone after ovulation and increase the power of GABA, a neurotransmitter that has a feel-good effect on our mood. In the majority of cisgender women, ALLO has a calming, antianxiety effect. However, in women with PMS and PMDD, ALLO can exacerbate negative moods. The thinking behind this contrasting effect is that the brain varies in sensitivity and in response to ALLO and progesterone. Some studies show that people with PMS have lower ALLO levels while other research shows that the levels of sex hormones don't significantly differ between people with PMS or PMDD and those without these conditions.

The ALLO paradox is one piece of the large and complicated puzzle when it comes to mood disorders during the luteal phase. Estrogen and its effects on serotonin are also implicated. Estrogen is necessary for the production and breakdown of serotonin, and it also increases serotonin receptor levels and sensitivity. A functioning serotonin system is important for memory, learning, and healthy mood. Estrogen enhances the functioning of our serotonin system, acting as a natural antidepressant when levels are high. When estrogen levels drop during the luteal phase, some of us who are especially sensitive to the effects of serotonin may experience extreme premenstrual mood symptoms. Because of their ability to increase serotonin activity, the standard treatment for severe PMS and PMDD is the class of antidepressant medication called selective serotonin reuptake inhibitors (SSRIs).

Interestingly, progesterone and ALLO are also implicated in motivation and addiction. During the luteal phase, studies show that cisgender women with high circulating progesterone who are addicted to cocaine experience lower blood pressure and report reduced anxiety and drug cravings compared to women with low circulating progesterone. A 2015 study out of *Psychoneuroendocrinology* looked at the effect of ALLO on stress response, drug cravings, and the ability of the individuals to inhibit their impulses and found that the group with high ALLO levels performed better in each of these categories. More ALLO was associated with positive emotions, an increased relaxed state, reduced drug cravings, and an improved ability to control impulsivity. Progesterone appears to reduce impulsive behavior via an increase in cognitive control, or our ability to be flexible, adaptable, and goal-directed in our thoughts and behaviors. What all of this means is that the luteal phase is an excellent time to create new habits and break old, destructive habits.

Reimagining Luteal

The luteal phase as a whole is the great balancer to the menstrual cycle. The late preovulatory and ovulatory phases are the highs of the menstrual cycle, when we feel really good and a bit more impulsive. The luteal phase is a time of grounding when we come back down to earth and firmly plant our feet on its surface. This time of heightened intentionality and connection is an opportunity to deeply examine and potentially change ingrained patterns. We've learned to pathologize our need for more self-care during this phase, blaming ourselves and our bodies for needing support and attention. But we can unlearn this blame and replace it with the understanding that support and self-care aren't signs of weakness or failure, but an essential part of our well-being.

This phase of inner autumn urges us to value the ongoing practice of care, or as the artist Mierle Laderman Ukeles refers to care, maintenance. In a 2009 interview, she described maintenance as "trying to listen to the hum of living. A feeling of being alive, breath to breath." As you deepen your attention and take care of yourself during the luteal phase, notice the hum of living all around you and within. Notice your breath, steadily maintaining your life, and the rise and fall of your hormones, maintaining the rhythm of your cycle and transitioning you once again to the beginning of a new season.

LET'S REVIEW
THE OVARIAN CYCLE

1. MENSTRUAL PHASE

- On day one of your cycle, you start bleeding because the corpus luteum regresses and estrogen and progesterone levels drop, triggering menstruation.

- Because of the low levels of estrogen and progesterone, the pituitary releases FSH (which actually gets released before you start your period).

2. PREOVULATORY PHASE

- Increasing FSH levels recruit ovarian follicles, which produce estrogen, increasing the amount of cervical mucus and encouraging the proliferation of the endometrium.

- One of the selected follicles becomes the dominant follicle and produces increasing amounts of estrogen. This peak in estrogen initiates the LH surge, which leads to the development of the corpus luteum.

- The preovulatory rise in progesterone occurs. Progesterone maintains the LH surge and is needed for the follicle to rupture from the ovary.

3. OVULATORY PHASE

- LH and progesterone, along with other compounds, degrade the wall of the ovary so that the dominant follicle can leave the ovary and travel into the fallopian tube, aka ovulation.

4. LUTEAL PHASE

- The corpus luteum is supported by LH and progesterone and secretes estrogen and progesterone.

- In the absence of fertilization, the corpus luteum starts to break down after six days and has an average lifespan of fourteen days.

- As the corpus luteum breaks down, decreasing progesterone and estrogen levels initiate menstruation. A new cycle begins.

WHY DO I WANT CHOCOLATE? EXPLAINING CRAVINGS

Before we get into the why of cravings, we need to acknowledge an important truth: chocolate isn't chocolate isn't chocolate. There's dark chocolate and milk chocolate, single origin, roasted and unroasted, sweetened with cane sugar versus alternative sweeteners, cacao powder and nibs, gritty bars and smooth bars, added flavors and straight-up. Chocolate is a spectrum of choice, and also importantly, not everyone chooses it.

A 2009 study from *Appetite* found that about half of American cisgender women crave chocolate, specifically at the onset of menstruation. The research was based on the premise that craving chocolate was related to premenstrual hormone changes. If craving chocolate was in fact related to sex hormones, postmenopausal women should experience a drop in their cravings. The study found a slight drop in postmenopausal women's chocolate cravings, but not one that was big enough to blame our desire for the sweet stuff on our sex hormones. The conclusion? Maybe chocolate cravings are a social or culture-bound construct of PMS, and maybe some people just like chocolate. But most likely, all of us are different and can't be lumped together into a premenstrual chocolate-craving generalized group.

CONTINUES

The concept of cravings is complicated. Among a wide range of languages, there is no equivalent translation of the word *craving*. Linguists tend to find that when a specific word in a particular language doesn't have a synonym in other languages, there is some doubt about the universality of the concept. In other words, in most non-English speaking countries, there isn't a word for "craving" because it isn't a universal phenomenon experienced by all people. In the 2009 *Appetite* study, the researchers found that when people from non-English-speaking countries are exposed to US culture, their likelihood of experiencing chocolate cravings around the time menstruation increases dramatically.

Cravings might be cultural, but changes in appetite during the menstrual cycle are physiological. During the follicular phase, our daily food intake tends to be lower than during the luteal and menstrual phases. Part of this appetite change is attributed to the complex web of hormones that impact our hunger and appetite. Cyclical changes in serotonin are associated with increased appetite, food cravings, and increased calorie intake in individuals with PMS and PMDD. Additionally, the way our bodies use nutrients from foods may be affected by the way our sex hormones change between phases. There is also some evidence that the menstrual cycle influences resting metabolic rate, with a higher rate in the luteal versus follicular phase. The research regarding appetite, cravings, and the menstrual cycle varies widely because studying appetite, which is both physiological and psychological, is inherently complex.

Whether it's cultural or biological or some combination, the appetite changes and cravings many people experience leading up to and during menstruation are real. Whether the desire is for chocolate, carbohydrates, protein, fats, sweets, salty food, or none of the above, we can treat ourselves gently and do our best to both enjoy food and eat mindfully.

Self-Care

Undercommit

There are two problems with overcommitment, defined as binding yourself to more than you can possibly accomplish. First, overcommitment leads to health issues including depression, diabetes, inflammatory diseases, cardiovascular disease, and sleep disorders. When we try to do too much, our body makes more stress hormones to help us cope with the added pressure. This contributes to an inflammatory state that weakens our immune system and encourages the development of chronic disease, which then disrupts the menstrual cycle and can cause more PMS symptoms and painful periods. The second problem with overcommitment has to do with the effort-reward imbalance theory. This theory builds on the idea that our efforts, or commitments, need to be appropriately compensated with either pay, opportunities, security, or recognition. When we're not rewarded for our efforts, our mental health suffers. We live in a culture of overcommitment and under-recognition where our efforts, especially if we are caring for children, are extremely high and also extremely under-rewarded. This combination is associated with emotional distress that can damage our health. During the luteal phase, practice saying no. Say no to the extra to-dos and unbind yourself from whatever commitments aren't absolutely essential.

Organize Your Nest

During the luteal phase, we may feel driven to organize, minimize, clean, and rearrange our homes. The nesting urge is an expression of our desire to control our environment and create a physically and emotionally safe space during times of unpredictability and transition. Cleaning and organizing may also help us cope with stress and anxiety. We are in a continual dialogue with our environment, adapting to changing circumstances and managing our energy. Situations that are unpredictable, complex, and uncontrollable provide us with an adaptative challenge and our instinct is to perform actions that help us regain a sense of control. This is known as the entropy model of uncertainty, and the repetitive, ritualistic, and predictable movements involved in cleaning and organizing help return us to a low-entropy state, therefore helping us manage stress and anxiety. During the transitions and shifts of the luteal phase, cleaning and nesting can act as therapy as we adapt to the changes happening within.

Dandelion-Infused Breast Oil and Breast Massage

Dandelion leaf is traditionally used in both Ayurveda and Traditional Chinese Medicine for breast health as it is rich in bioactive phytochemicals and contains potent antioxidants. Breast massage is a soothing self-care practice that increases circulation and lymphatic flow while also allowing you to assess your breasts for changes month to month. This oil was developed by the clinical herbalist Mary McCallum.

Makes 14 ounces, or enough for about 6 breast massages

2 ounces dried dandelion leaf

14 ounces extra virgin olive oil, sesame oil, almond oil, or apricot oil

Put the dandelion leaf in a blender and pulse until the leaf is broken down into a powder. Then put the powder in a 16-ounce mason jar and pour the oil over it. Tightly screw the lid on the jar and let the oil sit in a cool, dark space for 2 to 4 weeks, gently shaking the jar every few days to enhance the infusion process. Once the oil is infused, strain it into another mason jar and store it in a cool, dark place. Label the jar (include the date!) and use it within 6 months.

To give yourself a nourishing breast massage, place a small amount of the oil in your hands and warm it by rubbing your hands together. Gently rub the oil into your skin by making circles around your breast. This is best done in an upward and outward movement from the top of the breast to the armpit and then underneath the breasts circling toward the heart. Continue massaging around the breast, making sure you massage under your armpit and out toward your shoulders and upper chest.

Movement

During the first half of the luteal phase, energy levels remain high. So, if you're up to it, continue challenging yourself with increased natural movement and physical activity like you did during the ovulatory phase (see page 136). Mid-luteal, however, progesterone and estrogen levels begin to slowly decline to their lowest point, eventually triggering menstruation. During this transition, restorative movement such as walking and gentle restorative or yin yoga can feel really good. These kinds of meditative movements help improve the premenstrual experience by increasing blood flow, releasing endorphins, and offering anti-stress effects. A 2019 study compared the effectiveness of aerobic exercises like jogging versus vinyasa yoga in reducing the symptoms of PMS and found that while both types of movement practices had a positive effect on premenstrual symptoms, yoga was more effective in relieving negative PMS symptoms and decreasing pain intensity. The authors pointed out that yoga and aerobic exercises have similarities, but yoga emphasizes breathing control, intentionality, and peacefulness, which leads to a greater reduction in stress and anxiety.

Perceived stress or a negative perception of your health is significantly related to more painful and pronounced PMS symptoms before and during menstruation. That is, if you feel both unhealthy and stressed, you're more likely to experience premenstrual symptoms such as anxiety, mood swings, and depression. Fortunately, movement helps combat stress, and research shows that people who are physically active are more inspired to eat healthfully, which incidentally improves our health and importantly, makes us *feel* healthier. Along with walking and gentle yoga, here are a few more restorative movements that also reduce stress and set you up for a more positive premenstrual experience.

Roll It Out

Use a soft foam roller or therapy balls (also called fascia-release balls) to target sore spots and gently massage the body. A foam roller allows you to apply direct and sweeping pressure on your soft tissues, essentially providing you with a self-induced massage. One study showed that as compared to a non-foam-rolling group, rollers had reduced muscle soreness and were also more flexible and able to jump higher. Another study found that foam rolling enhanced recovery after exercise and subsequently improved performance measures such as sprint speed, dynamic strength, and endurance.

Start with gentle, long rolling strokes to help warm up the tissue and then spend some time targeting trigger points with slightly more pressure. A ten-minute rolling session is an efficient way to substantially boost muscle recovery and improve your ability to perform dynamic movements. Here are a few places to start rolling:

- Fronts and sides of the shins

- Calves

- Hamstrings

- Hip flexors and glutes

- Quadriceps and inner thighs

- Mid and upper back and between the shoulder blades

- Under the armpit along the rib cage

Move Your Eyes

Looking at screens or other up-close objects for long periods of time strains the eye muscles. Gazing into the distance is not only good for eye health but studies also show that walking in the woods or looking at trees and other green spaces outdoors reduces cortisol levels and stimulates the parasympathetic nervous system. Spending time outside in green spaces, urban or wild, improves our ability to recover from stress, supports relaxation, and boosts immune system health. Interestingly, unnatural images, especially those with striped patterns like stairs, buildings, and text, are measurably uncomfortable for our eyes to look at, especially for long periods of time, and cause an increase in oxygen uptake by the brain.

This oxygen uptake is meant to protect the brain as it uses more oxygen during times of visual discomfort. The bottom line? Spend more time outside looking at greenery and natural landscapes and take frequent breaks from looking at your computer or phone.

Take a Swing

One movement many of us don't get enough of is hanging and swinging with our arms over our heads. Find a sturdy tree branch or a pull-up bar and, keeping your shoulder blades down and engaged, pick up your feet for a short hang. Start with small durations, slowly building your grip strength and the muscle strength in your arms, back, and core. When you're ready, start swinging your legs, change up your grip and hand position, try the monkey bars, or climb some trees. Moving this way is like walking for the upper body. It gets our arms in a different position (overhead), which counteracts the way we usually use our arms (typing on a phone or computer) and improves shoulder stability and upper body strength. Importantly, hanging improves whole-body alignment and helps you breathe better. It also relieves and prevents lower back pain and lengthens, strengthens, and stretches your abdominal muscles and psoas.

Recipes

Kabocha Squash Curry Soup with Apples and Leeks

One of the most delicious and soothing meals to eat during fall, and our luteal phase, is winter squash soup. You can use a variety of different squashes for this recipe (butternut, acorn, or delicata as examples), but I love the earthy sweetness of kabocha and its beautiful dark green skin. This special squash is linked to improved blood sugar levels and digestive health and is also rich in vitamin C and antioxidants. Leeks and apples are excellent prebiotics, which provide nourishment to beneficial gut bacteria.

Makes 6 servings

1 large kabocha squash

2 tablespoons olive oil

1 large leek, thoroughly rinsed and thinly chopped

1 medium apple, cored and thinly sliced

Sea salt and fresh ground black pepper

2 tablespoons curry powder

½ teaspoon cayenne pepper

One 13.5-ounce can full-fat coconut milk

4 cups bone broth or vegetable broth

¼ cup plain full-fat yogurt, nondairy yogurt, buttermilk, or other cultured dairy product

TO SERVE, OPTIONAL

More cultured dairy of your choice

Fresh herbs (like parsley)

Avocado slices

Kimchi or sauerkraut

RECIPE CONTINUES

Preheat the oven to 400°F. Set the whole kabocha squash in a baking dish and roast until soft and easily pierced with a fork, about 1–1½ hours. Remove the squash from the oven, allow it to cool, then cut in half and scoop out the seeds.

Heat the olive oil in a large Dutch oven over medium heat. Add the leek and apple slices, season with salt and pepper, and let the mixture cook, stirring occasionally until the leeks are bright green and softened, around 5 to 7 minutes. Sprinkle in the curry powder and cayenne. Stir then spoon in the flesh from the kabocha squash, discarding the skin. Pour in the coconut milk and broth.

Transfer the soup to a tabletop blender (or use an immersion blender on the stovetop) and mix until smooth. Return the soup to the pot and bring it to a simmer. Taste and season generously with salt and pepper, then stir in the yogurt.

Ladle the soup into bowls and serve with the toppings of your choice.

Brothy Pureed White Beans with Pomegranate, Shallots, and Rainbow Chard

This recipe is inspired by a dish from Diana Henry's cookbook *A Change of Appetite*. She serves pureed beans with radicchio and red onions, which is utterly wonderful and highly recommended. But, since radicchio isn't always available, I enjoy using colorful rainbow chard or other leafy greens in its place and adding pomegranates and parsley for contrast and flavor. Beans are a great source of fiber and protein and they act as prebiotics, feeding our beneficial gut bacteria and supporting digestive health. This dish is like a hug for your insides and beautiful in its elegant simplicity. It is excellent served alongside roasted vegetables, fish, or crusty sourdough.

Makes 6 servings

1 cup dried or two 15-ounce cans cannellini beans

1 bay leaf

Olive oil

1 small onion or ½ large onion, chopped

1 garlic clove, crushed

½ cup bone broth or vegetable broth

Sea salt and pepper

Juice from 1 lemon, divided

3 shallots, thinly sliced

1 bunch chard or other leafy greens, chopped

1 bunch chopped parsley

Seeds from one pomegranate

Flaky sea salt

If using dried beans, put the beans in a large Dutch oven, cover with 2 inches of water, and soak for 8 to 12 hours. Drain the water from the beans then add fresh water, covering the beans by 1 inch. Add the bay leaf and bring the water to a boil over medium-high heat. Reduce the heat and simmer for 45 to 50 minutes, until the beans are tender. Drain the beans and discard the bay leaf.

RECIPE CONTINUES

Preheat the oven to 350°F. In a large cast iron skillet, heat 2 tablespoons of olive oil. Add the onion and cook until it is soft but not browned, then add the garlic, beans, broth, and a generous amount of salt and pepper. Stir everything together and cook for 5 minutes over medium heat.

Transfer the bean mix to a blender and add ¼ cup of olive oil and half the lemon juice. Blend until pureed and salt to taste. Transfer the beans into a medium oven-safe serving dish and place in the preheated oven until warmed through, about 15 minutes.

Add another 2 tablespoons of olive oil to a skillet and heat over medium-high heat. Add the shallots and quickly brown on both sides, then turn down the heat to medium-low and cook until the shallots are soft, 5 to 8 minutes. Add the chard to the pan, increasing the heat and cooking until wilted. Season with salt and pepper.

Pull the beans out of the oven. Top with the shallots and chard then sprinkle the parsley and pomegranates on top. Drizzle a little more olive oil on top along with a squeeze of lemon juice and a sprinkle of flaky sea salt.

Oven Braised Short Ribs

I love all of the meals in this book, but short ribs have a special place in my heart. They are delicious, comforting, and easy to prepare. This recipe is especially good served with winter squash and greens such as watercress or arugula. When you cook grass-fed beef on the bone until it is almost falling apart, you benefit from its high protein content, minerals, and vitamins along with glycine and collagen that becomes more bioavailable when you cook with bones, connective tissue, skin, and fat. Glycine nurtures gut and liver health and helps reduce systemic inflammation.

Makes 4–6 servings

2.5 pounds bone-in grass-fed beef short ribs, cut into single bone portions

2 tablespoons kosher salt

¼ cup shoyu, tamari, or coconut aminos

3 tablespoons sake

1 tablespoon coconut palm sugar

1 teaspoon miso

2-inch piece fresh ginger, grated

3 cloves garlic, minced

Olive or grapeseed oil

1 onion, chopped

1½ cups beef, chicken, or vegetable broth

TO SERVE

Lemon juice

Parsley

Plain full-fat yogurt

Season the short ribs with salt at least 1 hour before cooking or preferably overnight. If salting an hour before cooking, leave the ribs out on the counter so they come to room temperature. If salting the night before, store uncovered in the refrigerator, then remove and allow to come to room temperature an hour prior to cooking.

In a medium jar, combine the shoyu, sake, coconut palm sugar, miso, ginger, and garlic. Shake vigorously to combine.

Heat oven to 300°F. Heat 1½ tablespoons olive oil in a large Dutch oven over medium-high and add the short ribs, searing until brown on both sides, about 5 minutes a side. Transfer the ribs to a large plate and discard the excess fat (or save it for roasting vegetables).

Heat 1 tablespoon olive oil in the Dutch oven and add the onion, cooking over medium heat until the onion gets some color. Then pour the shoyu mixture into the pot, scape up the brown bits, and add the broth and the short ribs. Cover the pot and place in the oven for 3 hours. When ready, the ribs should be nearly fall-apart tender. Uncover, increase the oven to 425°F, and roast the ribs for another 30 to 40 minutes until nicely browned. Serve immediately with a squeeze of lemon juice, parsley, and a drizzle of yogurt.

Roasted Acorn Squash with Hazelnut Gremolata

This quintessential fall dish is both savory and sweet and also especially soothing during the luteal phase. Acorn squash is full of antioxidants, vitamin A, and vitamin C, and the cinnamon and cayenne pepper are warming spices. The hazelnut gremolata adds a crunchy dimension while the Greek yogurt adds essential balance.

Makes 4 servings

2 acorn squash (or delicata or butternut), cut in half, seeds removed (you can also remove the skin if you want, but I prefer to leave it on), and cut into 1-inch segments

Olive oil

½ teaspoon cinnamon

½ teaspoon cayenne pepper

Sea salt and freshly ground black pepper

TO SERVE

1 bunch spinach, mizuna, or other leafy green

Full-fat Greek yogurt

Olive oil

Lemon juice

Flaky sea salt

HAZELNUT GREMOLATA

⅓ cup hazelnuts or walnuts

½ lemon, zest and juice

2 garlic cloves

¼ cup olive oil

1 cup parsley leaves

1 teaspoon sea salt

Pepper

Preheat the oven to 400°F. Place the acorn squash on a parchment-lined or an unlined baking sheet, flesh side down. Drizzle generously with olive oil and sprinkle the cinnamon and cayenne on top. Season with sea salt and pepper. Roast the squash for 1 hour, flipping halfway through until both sides are browned and the squash is soft, sweet, and cooked all the way through.

While the squash roasts, make the gremolata. Spread the hazelnuts in a single layer on a dry, unlined baking sheet and roast them in the 400°F oven with the squash for about 5 minutes, then take them out and let cool slightly. Wrap them in a towel and rub vigorously to remove the skins. Add the hazelnuts, lemon zest and juice, garlic, olive oil, parsley, salt, and a grind of pepper to a food processor. Pulse until broken up but still chunky.

Place the spinach in a large serving bowl or into individual servings bowls. Spoon the roasted squash onto the greens, then place dollops of the gremolata on top, followed by several spoonfuls of yogurt. Finish with a drizzle of olive oil, lemon juice, and flaky sea salt.

Smashed Beets and Bitter Greens with Lemon Vinaigrette

Beets and bitter greens are rich in bioactive compounds and phytochemicals that provide health benefits including antioxidant and anti-inflammatory effects, vascular protection, and healthy liver function. Roasting and then smashing the beets maximizes their potential for crispiness while the acidity in the vinaigrette and bitterness of the greens balances out their earthy sweetness. ·

Makes 4 servings

3–4 medium-large beets, scrubbed and tough ends trimmed

Olive oil

Sea salt and freshly ground black pepper

1 bunch greens such as collards, kale, chard, mustard greens, dandelion, or other bitter greens (I like using a mix)

Fresh herbs such as cilantro or parsley, to serve

LEMON VINAIGRETTE

1 lemon, zest and juice

1 teaspoon raw honey

½ teaspoon sea salt

A few grinds of fresh cracked pepper

¼ cup olive oil

Preheat the oven to 425°F. Add the whole beets to a baking sheet lined with parchment paper, then roast them until fork-tender, 1 to 1½ hours depending on the size of your beets.

RECIPE CONTINUES

After cooling slightly, cut the beets into quarters and put them back on the baking sheet. Place another piece of parchment paper over the beets, and, using a cast iron skillet or some other heavy object, smash the beets until they are slightly flattened and round, like thick pancakes. Drizzle the beets with olive oil and season with plenty of salt and a grind of pepper. Place the beets back in the oven and roast until the beets and the skin are crispy, turning once and seasoning with more oil and salt, about 15 to 20 minutes.

While the beets roast, make the vinaigrette and prepare the greens. To make the vinaigrette, combine the lemon zest and lemon juice, honey, salt, pepper, and olive oil in a small mason jar and shake vigorously to combine. To prepare the greens, heat 2 tablespoons of olive oil in a large cast iron skillet over medium heat. Add the greens to the skillet, season with salt and sauté until wilted and some leaves are slightly browned and crisped.

To serve, spoon the greens into individual serving bowls and top with the crispy beets. Spoon vinaigrette over everything and serve with the fresh herbs of your choice.

Luteal Seed Balls

These nutty, complex, and just sweet enough luteal seed balls are packed with sesame seeds, which boast plentiful lignans and phytosterols, plant compounds that may lower cholesterol, along with vitamin E, calcium, and magnesium while sunflower seeds are also rich in vitamin E, vitamins B_1 and B_6, and iron, copper, selenium, and zinc. These are a good snack at any time of the month, but if you want to try seed cycling (see page 100), this recipe provides enough balls for the average luteal phase, starting on the day you ovulate and ending with the first day of your period. Consume one ball a day.

Makes 14 balls

½ cup tahini

1 tablespoon maple syrup

¼ cup melted coconut oil

¼ teaspoon sea salt

¾ cup raw sunflower seeds

¼ cup raw sesame seeds

½ cup unsweetened coconut flakes

¼ cup cacao nibs

2 pitted dates, finely chopped

In a small mixing bowl, whisk together the tahini, maple syrup, coconut oil, and salt. In a medium mixing bowl, stir together the sunflower seeds, sesame seeds, coconut flakes, cacao nibs, and dates. Stir the tahini mixture into the seed mixture until combined.

Using your hands or a cookie scoop, form the mixture into tablespoon-size balls and place them on a baking sheet lined with parchment or wax paper. Freeze until solid and then transfer the balls into an airtight container and put them back in the freezer. These will last for a month. When you're ready to enjoy one, allow the seed ball to come to room temperature for a few minutes before eating.

Roasted Pears with Maple Rosemary Walnuts and Greek Yogurt

This is an elegant dessert—not too sweet, a little savory—and the roasted maple rosemary walnuts fill your house with a smell I automatically associate with coziness and relaxation. I like to serve this with brunch or as an afternoon snack.

Makes 3 servings

3 pears, cored and halved

3 tablespoons lemon or orange juice

2 tablespoons maple syrup

4 tablespoons water

3 tablespoons unsalted butter

1 teaspoon vanilla extract

TO SERVE

Full-fat Greek yogurt

Cinnamon

MAPLE ROSEMARY WALNUTS

1 cup chopped walnuts

2 tablespoons unsalted butter

1 tablespoon maple syrup

1 tablespoon finely chopped rosemary

Zest from 1 lemon

Pinch of sea salt

Preheat the oven to 400°F. In a small saucepan, combine the lemon juice, maple syrup, water, butter, and vanilla and melt over low heat. Place the pears cut side down in a cast iron pan and pour the maple-syrup mix over the pears. Bake in the oven uncovered for 45 minutes.

While the pears bake, make the maple rosemary walnuts. Add the walnuts in a single layer on a baking sheet lined with parchment paper and roast them in the 400°F oven for 8 minutes. In the same small saucepan, combine the butter, maple syrup, rosemary, lemon zest, and salt. When the walnuts are done, use a rubber spatula to scrape the maple-butter mixture onto the walnuts and stir well to combine. Place the walnuts back in the oven and roast for another 8 minutes, stirring halfway through.

When the pears are done, spoon each pear into a bowl, top with the caramelized syrup, then dollop a few spoonfuls of the yogurt on top, followed by the maple rosemary walnuts and a sprinkle of cinnamon.

Chocolate Bark with Strawberries, Currants, and Toasted Coconut

Whatever the reason for chocolate cravings (see page 165), I'm down to eat some chocolate because it's delicious. I created this recipe when I wasn't eating any added sugar, but still wanted a delicious chocolate-y experience. The combination of freeze-dried strawberries, currants, and toasted coconut adds just enough sweetness and crunch to make this chocolate bark deeply satisfying. Cacao is rich in magnesium, potassium, iron, fiber, and flavonoids and aids in digestion, making this a perfect snack during the luteal phase.

Makes 4 servings

1 cup 100% cacao dark chocolate chips

2 tablespoons coconut oil

1 teaspoon vanilla extract

Pinch of sea salt

⅓ cup freeze-dried strawberries

¼ cup dried currants

¼ cup toasted coconut flakes

Set up a double boiler: in a small saucepan, bring 1–2 inches of water to a simmer, then place a glass bowl over the top so that it sits above—but not touching—the water. Add the chocolate chips and coconut oil and melt over medium-low heat for 5 to 8 minutes. Turn off the heat, then whisk in the vanilla and salt.

Carefully pour the chocolate onto a baking sheet lined with parchment paper, scraping out all the chocolate with a rubber spatula. Gently turn the pan side to side to create an even, thin chocolate layer. Evenly sprinkle the freeze-dried strawberries, currants, and coconut flakes over the chocolate then place in the refrigerator until set (about an hour). Break the bark into pieces and store it in an airtight container in the fridge for up to a week.

Maple Pear Custard

This quick, classy dessert is adapted from a Martha Stewart pear custard pie recipe that I first made for a close friend and subsequently adapted to contain less sugar and more cream and eggs. This custard is rich in fat and protein from the cream and eggs as well as fiber from the pears, which helps prevent sugar highs (and subsequent crashes) that often follow eating sweet treats. Choose pears that are just ripe, not too firm, and not too soft.

Makes 6 servings

3 pears, cored, halved, and sliced into ¼-inch slices

4 eggs

¾ cup cream (grass-fed dairy or coconut cream)

⅓ cup almond flour

2 tablespoons maple syrup

1 teaspoon vanilla extract or ¼ teaspoon vanilla powder

¼ teaspoon sea salt

¼ cup unsalted butter, melted

Preheat the oven to 350°F.

Butter a 9-inch pie dish and arrange the pear slices in a circle on the bottom so that they overlap.

In a medium bowl, whisk together the eggs, cream, almond flour, maple syrup, vanilla, sea salt, and butter until thoroughly combined. Alternatively, you can blend these ingredients in a blender. Pour the batter over the pears and then bake until golden, about 40 to 45 minutes. Serve on its own, or with plain Greek yogurt or freshly whipped cream.

Nourishing Blood-Building Tea

Jujube dates and goji berries are traditionally used by Chinese medicine to support blood-building. Nettle leaf, which is rich in vitamins and minerals, is balanced by the flavors of citrus peel, ginger, and anise. This is a complex, deeply nourishing tea developed by the clinical herbalist Mary McCallum to enjoy during the late luteal or menstrual phase. All of the herbs in this recipe are available to order online, but if you can't find all the herbs in this recipe, or only want to buy a few to try, no worries. As with all recipes, use what you have and adapt. For example, you could use fennel seeds in place of the anise, or regular Medjool dates instead of jujube dates.

Makes 2 servings

4 cups water

2 jujube dates, pits removed

2 tablespoons goji berries

2 tablespoons nettle leaf

1 tablespoon citrus peel

1 tablespoon anise seed

½ teaspoon ground ginger

In a medium saucepan, add all the ingredients and simmer covered for 15 to 20 minutes. Strain the herbs using a fine mesh strainer or cheesecloth into a 32-ounce mason jar and sip this tea throughout the day. Store the tea in a thermos so it stays warm.

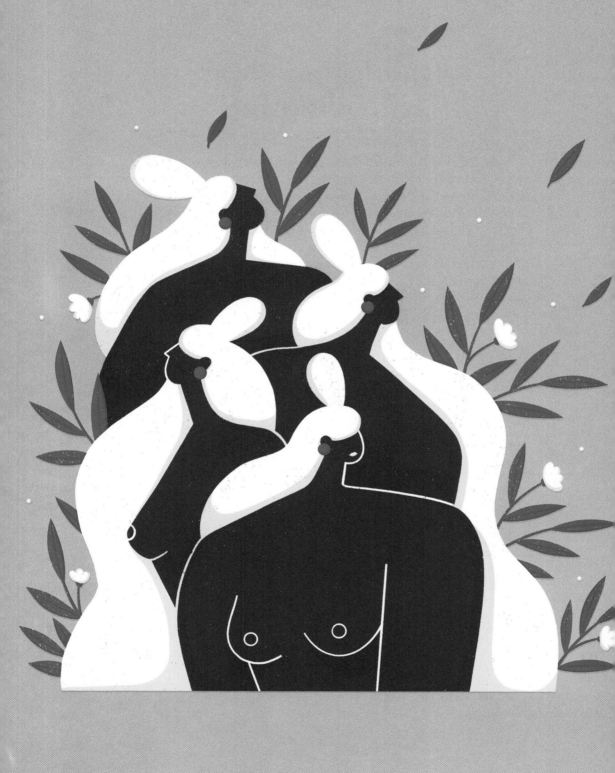

PART THREE

Exploring the Four Seasons of Life

In parts one and two, we've explored the seasonality of the menstrual cycle phases, but now let's turn toward the seasonality of life. From menarche [the establishment of menstruation] to the menstruating years to the menopausal transition and postmenopause, Part Three explores where we've been, where we are, and where we're headed. The purpose of these chapters is to highlight the most significant factors that impact overall and reproductive health during each season of life. We are born as one form and change slowly, but constantly. How we navigate those changes matters because those choices come together to make our life.

When we're in one season of life, it's rare to think about the next season, and there is not much substantial education on these phases. We get a mediocre lesson about menstrual cycles during our adolescence, but most of us don't sit down in a classroom and learn in-depth about what will happen. During what is considered the reproductive years, the menopausal transition feels so far away; it's something we either never think about or barely consider. Then, when we're on the brink of the menopausal transition, we might mourn or even dread the change. By highlighting what you can expect in each season of life, I hope these chapters will give you the confidence to navigate, and even celebrate, these changes. The goal is to provide you with greater knowledge and tools so that as you enter a new season, you're not caught off guard by the weather.

Menarche

AGE ±12–18

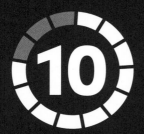

My seventh-grade health class teacher called sex "wrestling." Every time the word was about to come up in a lecture, he would turn red, cough awkwardly, and turn his hands into giant quotation marks so that we understood that he was not actually talking about wrestling. This embarrassed man was, incidentally, the wrestling coach, and he'd been tasked with teaching a subject to middle schoolers that he was clearly not prepared for. There are obvious problems with replacing "sex" with "wrestling." For one, while you should protect yourself when either having sex or wrestling, only one of these activities can result in pregnancy. For another, wrestling is a stereotypically masculine sport that involves domination and pinning, which is obviously problematic when teaching the importance of respect and consent.

At the time, cringing in embarrassment, I didn't fully understand why I felt so uncomfortable that my teacher, who was also clearly uncomfortable, was incapable of using the right words to talk about the human body and reproductive health. Now, I understand that language shapes our understanding of the world around us and ourselves and clear language from qualified and confident teachers helps us build a frame for that understanding. Part of the reason I felt so uncomfortable was because, on some level, I realized that he was part of a larger narrative that was shaping how we thought about sex. Told the wrong way, the normal becomes shameful and our bodies and their functions become embarrassing instead of empowering. Further, the use of euphemisms can lead to a misrepresentation of meaning, which then creates misunderstanding of what something actually is. "Wrestling," the verb, as a stand-in for the most important and consequential reproductive act humans take part in, might be funny if the consequences weren't so high.

You might have a similar story from your adolescence and remember cringing in health class while someone talked about subjects that felt private and personal—like periods and sex—in a way that was uncomfortable or embarrassing. Maybe, like me, you remember the boys acting horrified about periods and childbirth, and this social disapproval led to the first feelings of shame about your body and its functions. Whatever experience you had—good, bad, or neutral—it influenced and continues to influence your self-concept and ingrained beliefs about menstruation and sexuality. What we learn about sexuality and our bodies during adolescence matters because our psychosocial competencies—including self-esteem, emotional and moral competence, and resilience—influence the kinds of choices we make.

Sexual behavior is especially influenced by these competencies. In a 2019 review about sex education in different countries, the authors found that most school-based sex education is "home-baked," meaning each school comes up with its own style of educating about sex that, in general, lacks a theoretical framework and robust research. These programs are often created by policymakers who aren't directly involved in sex education or research about sex education and then taught by teachers who aren't specially trained or especially passionate about teaching adolescents about sex. The result is a highly variable, questionably effective, arguably lackluster sexual education that leaves out the major factors that underlie adolescent sexuality including anatomical, hormonal, physical, cognitive, social, cultural, and physiological dimensions.

THE CONDOM QUEEN

In 1993, Joycelyn Elders became the first Black and the second woman to be named US surgeon general. She fought for comprehensive health and sex education in schools, bringing up taboo topics like condom use to prevent teen pregnancy and HIV/AIDS, and, famously, masturbation. In 1994, she was asked to resign after she made a comment that masturbation is a part of human sexuality and should perhaps be talked about and taught in schools. In a 2021 interview with Wendy Zukerman on the podcast "Science Vs," Elders, 88 years old at the time of the recording, said of masturbation, "It won't make you go crazy. It won't make you go blind. And you know you're having sex with somebody you love."

During her time as surgeon general, she was condemned by religious conservatives and referred to as "The Condom Queen" as she promoted safe sex and passed out free condoms through the Health Department. She even had a condom tree on her desk and said of her nickname, "If I could be the 'condom queen' and get every young person who engaged in sex to use a condom in the United States, I would wear a crown on my head with a condom on it!" She continued advocating for better sex ed in schools, including distributing contraception, teaching about masturbation, and promoting health and racial equality, as a professor of pediatrics at the University of Arkansas for Medical Sciences. Elders was ahead of her time, but many states still require teaching abstinence in sex ed, and the US continues to have higher rates of teen pregnancy compared to similar countries. All of this to say the remarkable and revolutionary advocacy from the Condom Queen, Joycelyn Elders, is just as relevant today as it was in the 1990s.

The intersection of menstruation, reproduction, and sexuality is often not articulated during adolescence, which leaves gaps in our understanding of our own biology. Further, adolescents are bombarded with different opinions from pop culture, peers, and adults about what the menstrual cycle symbolically means. As Elizabeth Kissling, a writer, applied linguist, and professor of gender, women's studies, and sexuality at Eastern Washington University, put it, "Girls in the USA receive mixed messages about menarche: menarche is traumatic and upsetting—but act normal; menarche is an overt symbol of sexual maturity—but also a mysterious, secret event." This dualistic messaging about our reproductive functioning creates internal conflict that can promote lasting shame about our bodies and affect sexual decision-making and overall self-concept.

Better Sex Ed

If you're a parent, coach, teacher, mentor, friend, or family member of a young person learning about menstruation, you might be wondering how to model body positivity and reduce menstrual stigma and shame. To do this, it helps to understand puberty and what is going on in the body and brains of young people who are going through this major life transition. So, first, let's look at the basic biology of puberty and the brain changes that accompany it, then we can talk about how to resist and reduce menstrual shame.

Puberty and the Gut-Brain-Stress Connection

On average, the first period shows up at around twelve-and-a-half years old, or around two-and-a-half years after a girl first starts growing breasts, which may happen anywhere from ages six to thirteen (not including early or late puberty). While we don't know the exact mechanism that controls the timing of puberty, we do know that gonadotropin-releasing hormone (GnRH) is responsible for initiating the menstrual cycle once puberty gets rolling. Imagine the brain suddenly lighting up as neurons in the hypothalamus start releasing GnRH in pulses that signal the anterior pituitary to increase its release of the hormones FSH and LH. Next, the hormones released from the brain travel to the ovaries and tell them to wake up. FSH tells the ovaries to release more estrogen, and LH initiates ovulation and creates the corpus luteum, entering the body into the luteal phase. Then, dropping levels of estrogen and progesterone trigger the first menstruation, also known as menarche. The brain and ovaries are now communicating, responding to each other's signals. This rhythmic connection (the menstrual cycle) is considered the culmination of puberty for people who menstruate and the physiologic shift that takes the body to the next level of physical maturity where we gain the capacity to procreate.

Along with breast development and menstruation, the adrenal glands start pumping out increased hormone levels (which encourages pubic and armpit hair growth and can contribute to acne). Prompted by increasing estrogen levels and growth hormone, most people grow taller (which is also influenced by genetics and environmental factors such as nutrition). The vagina, clitoris, and other external genitalia enlarge; vaginal secretions increase; and the vaginal pH becomes more acidic about a year before menarche.

In addition to these observable physical changes, adolescents going through puberty undergo significant physiological changes in the brain. The first episodes of psychiatric disorders such as anxiety, depression, and eating disorders tend to appear, on average, around age fifteen. One of the reasons researchers believe these disorders emerge during adolescence is because the most ubiquitous stressors of adolescence, including a poor diet, not enough sleep, social stress, and drug and alcohol use, have a negative effect on brain development and gut microbiota. Research is starting to explore the relationship between the gut microbiome and the stress response, and evidence suggests that the microbes that inhabit the gut during childhood and adolescence have a lasting effect on stress circuitry— or how the brain perceives and responds to stress in the long run.

Puberty is a conduit toward future independence, but we never escape the dependence we have on our microbiome and its undeniable role in shaping our health. The self-care, movement practices, and foods recommended at the end of this chapter (see page 196) are specifically geared to nurture the diversity and health of the intestinal microbiota and help promote a more adaptable and resilient stress circuit in the brain. These offerings are adapted for you to share with adolescents in your life, but really, they are applicable and useful at any age.

Resisting Shame

How we come to know ourselves and whether or not we experience a negative, self-critical mindset is mediated through our concept of self and our relationship to our bodies. The menstrual cycle is a formative experience for our body-self relationship, and it is helpful to remember this when we consider adolescents learning about and experiencing menstruation for the first time. How people feel about menstruation is molded by the messages they take in about periods from culture, teachers, family, and friends. Before experiencing their first period, research shows that girls already believe that the event will be physically uncomfortable with heightened emotionality and negative mood changes. When menstruation happens, girls' conversations with other people who menstruate tend to focus on the bad parts, like period cramps and pain. Negative messaging about the menstrual cycle combined with communication that highlights bad experiences creates a disempowering social construct of menstruation. This construct is then perpetuated and reinforced by social media and advertising that represent periods as undesirable roadblocks to success and joy. The result of this social perception of menstruation as something bad that needs concealing is shame about this bodily process, and period shaming is still a common experience.

Shame is like an invasive weed. It starts with a feeling that the menstrual cycle is something dirty and embarrassing and spreads to a belief that the body itself is shameful. When we feel this way about our bodies, we're more likely to also feel this way about other people's bodies (no matter their gender) and about reproductive functions such as pregnancy, childbirth, and breastfeeding. And there is a cost: low self-esteem, high body shame, increased effort taken to conceal menstruation, and poorer sexual decision-making are all consequences of feeling embarrassed by our bodily functions.

A 2005 study in the *Journal of Sex Research* investigated the relationship between menstrual shame and whole-body shame among 199 undergraduate cisgender women. The authors hypothesized that since girls often learn about menstruation and sex at the same time—at home and/or in health class—their attitudes about both are connected and affect sexual decision-making. They found that menstrual cycle shame is associated with sexual decision-making via body shame. Cis women who reported feeling more menstrual cycle shame were more likely to be less sexually active, *but* take more sexual risks, whereas those who reported more comfort with menstruation were also more comfortable in their bodies, more sexually assertive, and sexually experienced, but they took less sexual risks.

Therefore, reducing menstrual shame has the capacity to improve overall body image and positively support sexual agency.

So how do we build confidence and fight against period stigma? That depends on who you are and what your skill set is. Some people make beautiful art with their menstrual blood; Kiran Gandhi, the drummer, activist, and artist, choose to free bleed during a marathon, demonstrating that her period wasn't going to stop her from participating in the event. Other activists fight for menstrual equality and menstrual product accessibility through research, lobbying, working with lawmakers, writing, social media, movies, and advertisements. Menstrual activism doesn't have to start with grand gestures. You can start by acknowledging that menstrual cycle shame and stigma are real and the consequences are negative for all people. You can start by assessing how the way you feel about your cycle has affected you and then teach the people who are close to you who menstruate—like your children—that the menstrual cycle isn't shameful or embarrassing.

When I was younger, I taught outdoor science education. On a five-day backpacking and field science trip, one of the young girls in my group started her period for the first time. The other teachers looked at me like, *There is no way we are doing this*, so I got a baggy full of menstrual products and found a private place among these huge backcountry boulders where I could help her. She was clearly scared and unprepared, so I told her that I get my period too, that it's healthy, and I was there to help her with whatever she needed. This gesture of normalcy, empathy, understanding, and support is what all people who menstruate deserve.

Dr. Inga Winkler, coeditor of *The Palgrave Handbook of Critical Menstruation Studies*, says that we need early, age-appropriate education about the menstrual cycle so that we know if we're experiencing a normal menstrual cycle or if we need to seek medical attention. By talking about PMS and cramps and not hiding the bleeding phase from young people, we normalize the menstrual experience. In taking these steps, we advocate for agency and autonomy and a culture that allows menstruators to make their own decisions about their bodies. Together, we can resist patriarchal messages that menstruation is shameful, unclean, and unfeminine and change the script. When we can approach our cycles with confidence and dignity, we find the key to empowerment and self-advocacy. The lesson that we are worthy of honor, respect, and gender equality is perhaps the most profound and important lesson we can learn at any age in our lives.

THE BACKPACK KIT

If you're a parent or if you work with people who may soon menstruate
for the first time, this is the ultimate teaching and preparedness kit.
It can go with adolescents on the verge of menarche or those who
are already cycling, to camps, sleepovers, school, and even their first
backpacking trip. Put it together with your child or carry it with you if
you're a teacher and you won't be caught off guard by this new season
of life. Many companies offer kits for new or seasoned menstruators. You
can purchase one or make your own with the items listed below. While
this kit is helpful for new menstruators, I bring it with me on camping,
climbing, and multiday skiing and backpacking trips.

- Waterproof pouch to store everything.

- Menstrual products: you can adjust this based on your needs, but to
  cover all the bases, consider packing 8 reusable or disposable pads
  (4 heavy, 4 regular), 2 pairs of period underwear, a small box of
  tampons, or a menstrual cup if desired.

- Reusable silicone bag for used products.

- Non-toxic hand sanitizer: soap and water are best for handwashing,
  but hand sanitizers are the next best on-the-go option.

- Extra credit: A notebook and pen to track your cycle and sustainable
  menstrual products.

- Supplements (optional): Some companies make safe, tasty vitamins
  and elixirs that are intended to naturally relieve cycle-related
  symptoms such as stress, cramping, bloating, and anxiety.

Self-Care and Movement

No matter what stage of life you're in, the following self-care and movement practices are beneficial and support overall health. That said, these suggestions are tailored specifically toward adolescents because they are especially susceptible to mental health distress from social media use, and they need their parents, teachers, and mentors to model healthy living by going outside often and moving their bodies in many different ways.

Disconnect

More than two hours a day of screen time is associated with poorer mental health among teenagers, including lower levels of optimism and satisfaction in life and higher anxiety and depressive symptoms. Between 2010 and 2015, depressive symptoms and suicide rates increased, in particular among adolescent females. Data has connected this increase to screen time—the more time teenagers spend on their phones, the more likely they are to experience adverse mental health effects, which could have an outcome related to suicide, such as making a suicide plan. The toxicity of devices is no joke. It's a huge issue, as more than half of the US teenage population spends more than five hours a day on an electronic device.

Okay, so what do we do? One study showed that adolescents who spend more time on nonscreen activities like sports, exercise, in-person social interaction, print media, religious services, and homework are less likely to report mental health problems. In addition to increasing nonscreen activities, we can also create healthier boundaries for all family members such as eliminating the use of devices during meals, keeping devices out of bedrooms at night, and creating rules about where, when, and how screens can be used and for how long.

Connect

Our happiness, well-being, and health are directly connected to how much time we spend outside, specifically in natural environments such as parks, forests, and beaches. A 2019 study in *Scientific Reports* found that spending at least 120 minutes in contact with natural places each week is associated with consistently higher levels of well-being and health. Instilling the love of nature in children is the best way to create a habit that gets them up and outside for the rest of their lives. A couple of ways to increase outside time include walking a dog (if you have one); growing a garden if you have space (even a few pots outside or a window planter will do!); cooking outside; going outside for activities such as biking, hiking, swimming, and camping; and attending nature-based or wilderness camps. Fostering a connection to nature is an essential part of living well and joyfully as a human being, and it is our responsibility to nurture our adolescents' connection to the natural world.

Diversify Your Sports

An increasing trend among young, developing athletes is early specialization in sports. Intense, year-round, sport-specific training is associated with overuse injury from repetitive movements that stress the same musculoskeletal tissues over and over again. A 2019 study in *Frontiers in Pediatrics* found that adolescent cisgender females who specialized in a sport were at higher risk for knee injuries compared to multisport female athletes. What we need at a young age—and throughout our lives—is variable and diverse movements that improve motor function and neuromuscular control. Participating in many sports and physical activities allows for improved physical and motor development. Further, while our culture enforces the idea that specialization is a key part of achievement, there is no evidence that specializing in a sport early on results in greater success. Balance out participating in multiple sports with plenty of play and unstructured activities to ensure dynamic strength and movement.

Get Creative

Sports aren't the only pathway to full-body movement. Plant a garden, try rock climbing, incorporate movement breaks into your routine, learn how to forage for wild food, or practice different kinds of dance. Create obstacle courses outside, climb trees, learn to build furniture, or cook meals from scratch over a fire that you build. Set up life in a way that requires more daily, whole body, natural movement.

MENARCHE
Nutrition

The most rapid growth and development occur when we're babies and during puberty. Research shows that a healthy diet may help reduce the ill effects of social stress that lead to increased problems with memory, mood, and cognitive function among adolescents. Along with consuming diverse, whole foods, it is essential to nourish healthy eating habits during this phase. A few nutrients that are especially important for adolescents include iron, choline, chromium, folate, vitamin A, E, B_6, calcium, zinc, magnesium, and fiber. Adequate protein and healthy fats are also essential. Below, we'll dive into iron and DHA; however, the best way to get the body what it needs is to eat a wide variety of fruits, vegetables, fermented foods, seafood, pastured meats and eggs, and of course, to drink plenty of water.

Iron

Iron deficiency is extremely common, especially among menstruating adolescents. We need adequate iron stores to support hemoglobin production, immune function, cognitive development, energy metabolism, and temperature regulation. The most absorbable form of iron is heme iron in meat (compared to non-heme iron in both meat and plants). Adequate intestinal absorption of iron requires a healthy digestive system and adequate levels of vitamin B_{12} and folate. Vitamin C enhances iron absorption, while calcium-rich foods such as milk and yogurt inhibit it.

Iron-rich foods include meats and stews made with bones, organ meats like chicken and beef liver, and seafood (especially clams, mussels, and oysters). A few vitamin C–rich foods are citrus fruits, strawberries, papaya, peppers, tomatoes, broccoli, cantaloupe, and chard. Cooking in cast iron cookware increases the iron content of food. Non-heme iron can be found in nuts, pumpkin, sesame, hemp and flaxseeds, whole grains, legumes, beans, and vegetables.

Omega-3 Fatty Acids

The long-chain omega-3 fatty acid, DHA (docosahexaenoic acid), supports brain health as a structural component of brain cells, memory, and cognitive development. Some studies show that eating a lot of fish, which is rich in omega-3s and DHA, is protective against the development of major depressive disorder, especially in cisgender females. The best food sources include fish and other seafood, particularly cold-water fish such as salmon, anchovies, mackerel, tuna, sardines, and herring. Fish eggs, oysters, halibut, trout, grass-fed beef, and eggs from pasture-raised chickens are also rich in DHA, while flaxseeds, walnuts, hempseeds, and chia seeds are good sources of omega-3s, but not DHA. Aim to consume these foods throughout the week, and you can also supplement with fish oil with at least 300 mg/day DHA.

Positive Body Image and Healthy Eating Patterns

Studies show that cisgender girls are more likely to report dissatisfaction with their weight and appearance. During puberty, worries about body image may be acute, and some of the consequences of an unhealthy body image include low self-esteem, eating disorders, and mental health disorders such as depression. Cultivate body positivity and healthy eating habits by modeling these traits. Children whose parents' express dissatisfaction with their bodies are more likely to have negative body image. Even if you don't have children, modeling body positivity can be beneficial for younger people in your life—and it's good for you too! Focus on appreciating the body for what it can do versus how it looks. Celebrate food and make healthy eating a part of your life, and avoid criticizing others—and yourself—based on weight or appearance.

The Menstruating Years

AGE ±12–51

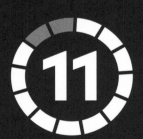

11

Jane Catherine Severn, a psychotherapist from New Zealand coined the word *menstruality* in 2004 because she felt that people with ovaries didn't have a word to describe what she called the "4 M's": menarche, menstruation, menopause, and the mature years. Menstruality encompasses the process of evolving and the knowledge gained along the way and thus is a broad and multidimensional word for the growth that occurs physiologically, psychologically, and spiritually from menarche through the years of menstruation, menopause, and finally, the postmenopausal years. Part of that growth includes learning how to deeply pay attention to and care for ourselves in a world that rarely prioritizes our cyclic health. Menstruality is a process of ownership and acceptance, and importantly, it is a journey of discovering what works for you.

During our menstruating years, we're introduced to competing demands on our attention as we navigate decisions about our careers, partners, whether or not we want to have children, and, if we do want to have children, when and how many? These choices pull us in multiple directions as we consider choices and requirements of our time, energy, relationships, and finances that are incredibly stressful and easily show up as tension in our bodies or as other health problems. In the early reproductive years, the menstrual cycle may settle into a somewhat predictable, and this sweet time of our young adult lives is marked by possibility and exploration, where anything and everything seems possible. At some point, especially if we've chosen to raise children, our lives are shaped more by responsibility and an extension of ourselves to the service and care of others. While fulfilling and meaningful, this period is also marked by what the writer, feminist, and activist Caroline Criado Perez calls the unpaid care burden. In her book *Invisible Women*, she writes that women do 75 percent of the world's unpaid care. For example, grocery shopping, housecleaning, and dropping the kids off at school. The unpaid and paid labor of women is the backbone of our society and economy. This labor is undervalued and often uncompensated, and the price we pay for this inequality is often our physical and emotional health and safety.

In this chapter, we'll focus on a few major health challenges we often face during our menstruating years and how to improve our resilience and thus our journey through menstruality. Specifically, we'll examine the relationship between burnout and fertility and how chronic stress leads to abnormal cortisol rhythms and levels. Then, we'll talk about how to build our resilience and resistance to burnout and chronic stress. First, let's explore an issue that is made worse by gender inequality and has negative consequences for our overall health: burnout syndrome.

Burnout Syndrome

Burnout is the word used to describe a specific kind of relentless exhaustion that damages our health and well-being. The traditional definition of burnout syndrome includes three dimensions: a reduced sense of personal accomplishment, depersonalization of others, and emotional exhaustion. A few components that determine the development of burnout syndrome include heavy workload, lack of control, the feeling that we aren't adequately rewarded for our work, the need to do more for less compensation, impersonal communities that lack teamwork, unfair conditions, and conflicting values between management and workers. While burnout is studied in relationship to working environments, it's easy to see many of the components of burnout showing up in all corners of our lives, whether at work, in the home, or other places where we experience the unpaid care burden. There are numerous health consequences of burnout—depression, cardiovascular disease, musculoskeletal pain, and sleep disorders to name a few.

Some studies also find a relationship between burnout and fertility. A 2014 study out of Hungary about the correlation between reproductive disorders and burnout among female physicians found that burnout is an important risk factor for miscarriages and high-risk pregnancies, and it negatively affects pregnancy outcomes. Other research finds that when cisgender women perceive their work as more demanding, they are less likely to conceive after receiving fertility treatments. Meanwhile, working fewer hours is associated with a higher likelihood of conception.

In 1987, the Mind/Body Program for Fertility started teaching infertility patients relaxation techniques and education about lifestyle changes and social support. The program also offers a form of psychotherapy called cognitive behavioral therapy (CBT). CBT is meant to rewire our thought patterns, cultivating self-awareness and challenging self-blame and other damaging thoughts. CBT is not specifically for people struggling with infertility. It is a type of talk therapy used to treat a wide range of conditions including depression, anxiety, OCD, and eating disorders among other mental health struggles. By combining lifestyle guidance with mental health support, The Mind/Body Program for Fertility has proven itself as a powerful intervention for people struggling with infertility as it successfully lowers stress *and* increases pregnancy rates. The program is one of the more compelling examples that psychological interventions affect reproductive health.

While lifestyle influences whether or not we develop burnout, it's essential to point out that burnout is not a personal failure. If we're burned out, it's not because we didn't meditate enough, eat the right foods, or move our bodies enough. These actions help improve our resilience, but burnout is more often the result of systemic and/or racial and gender inequality and dismal social support for parents and nonparents alike. For example, if you do decide to have a child and live in the United States, you are living in the only industrialized country that doesn't guarantee workers paid maternity or paternity leave. In fact, 85 percent of people in the United States who have babies are not offered any form of paid leave. Not only do we lack parental leave, but we also lack affordable childcare options, meaning that if and when we decide to return to work, we must pay someone else a lot of money to watch our children. This increases the risk of burnout and the stress that comes with it and is often an insidious and lonely struggle that leads to heightened anxiety and self-blame. Constant strains on our time and emotional and physical energy contribute to chronic stress. In the next section, we'll look at how chronic stress leads to abnormal cortisol levels or rhythms.

The Highs and Lows of Cortisol

Normal cortisol levels rise in the morning, helping us wake up with energy and clarity, and decrease as the day passes, following a circadian rhythm that facilitates various processes in the body, like cellular repair. When we experience a threat to our well-being, a chain of endocrine events is triggered that results in the release of epinephrine, norepinephrine, and cortisol from the adrenal glands. These adaptive hormones give us a survival edge, increasing blood sugar, decreasing sensitivity to pain, bolstering immune resistance, and boosting our energy and focus. Cortisol levels peak about fifteen to twenty minutes after the onset of stress, and its job is to decrease inflammation, mobilize glucose for energy, and suppress nonvital organ systems. After the stress from a threat has resolved, stress hormones should eventually drop back down to their baseline levels.

When cortisol remains elevated after an acute stress event, the effects are disastrous. The result includes symptoms such as fatigue, depression, memory impairment, and bone and muscle breakdown. Chronic stress is also associated with cognitive inflexibility and poor coping skills. With poor coping skills, we become more sensitive to stressors and experience a heightened physiologic stress response. This response is due to cortisol-induced memory formation whereby increased cortisol levels cause our brain to interpret stressors as threatening and frightening and then release more cortisol in response to future stressors. This chronic reactivation of the stress response is tiring, and the resulting cortisol dysregulation is linked to chronic fatigue, inflammation, and pelvic pain, among other diseases.

Under chronic stress, the hypothalamus-pituitary-adrenal (HPA) axis is initially hyperactive and we experience high levels of cortisol. But it may then become less active, or hypoactive, with low levels of cortisol. Studies have shown that chronic pain, anxiety, and depression are associated with low cortisol levels and a flattened or suppressed cortisol diurnal rhythm, meaning less of a cortisol peak in the morning when we need energy and less of a drop in the evening when we need sleep. One study showed that for cisgender women, a disrupted cortisol rhythm is significantly associated with increased pain sensitivity and musculoskeletal pain. The cognitive and physical effects of stress and pain are especially visible in conditions like endometriosis. Pelvic pain is the most common symptom of endometriosis, and people with this condition tend to have more concerns about their fertility. This fertility stress leads to increased anxiety and what's called "pain catastrophizing," or a heightened response to anticipated pain, which then increases and amplifies painful experiences. Further, if this pain disrupts relationships, self-esteem and social supports are damaged, which even further worsens pain.

Chronic stress is a vicious cycle, but it's not a trap. Physical and psychological interventions that reduce stress and normalize cortisol levels and rhythms have the potential to reduce or relieve many of the symptoms of cortisol dysfunction. In a study in the *Journal of Psychosomatic Obstetrics & Gynecology*, cisgender women with endometriosis and chronic pelvic pain underwent physical and psychological therapy once a week for ten weeks and had their salivary cortisol levels drawn three times a day. At the end of the treatment protocol, the individuals reported lower perceived stress and higher vitality and physical functioning. Cortisol levels were higher in the samples collected in the morning, but not in the samples collected in the afternoon or evening. This study demonstrates the possibility for change and how the actions we take have the capacity to restore our health and reduce chronic stress and pain.

Complete the Cycle

Building resilience and resistance to burnout and chronic stress starts with identifying that we're burned out and stressed. Feeling consistently physically and emotionally exhausted; more negative, detached, and cynical; and like your work is ineffective and unimportant are key signs of burnout. Because both burnout and chronic stress slowly develop over time, it can be challenging to identify these crises and difficult to change the circumstances that led to them in the first place. Awareness is the first step to resilience. Of awareness and attention, the late American author and essayist Barry Lopez wrote, "Perhaps the first rule of everything we endeavor to do is to pay attention. Perhaps the second is to be patient. And perhaps the third is to be attentive to what the body knows." When it comes to addressing chronic stress and burnout, start with attention, follow up with patience—with yourself and with the circumstances—and allow your body to do what it knows. One thing the body instinctively knows is how to complete a stress cycle.

In their book *Burnout: The Secrets to Unlocking the Stress Cycle*, sisters Emily and Amelia Nagoski write about actions that complete the stress cycle. The stress cycle is the event of experiencing a threat to our survival and the actions that follow. We're out in the world, an animal almost eats us, but we run away, survive, take deep, relieving breaths, and, in a gathering with our friends, we celebrate that we survived. These steps—running away, breathing, socializing, and gratitude—are all key parts of completing the stress cycle. The single most effective way to complete the stress cycle, the authors write, is physical activity. When we are in motion, we inherently and physically understand that we're fully alive. As you'll read in the "Find a Walking Buddy" section on page 208, moving is the embodiment of forward progress. In the case of stress, locomotion physically and mentally moves us away from that stress and toward a sense of peace and well-being. Breathing is another way to complete the stress cycle. When deeply and slowly performed, our breath tells our brain it's okay, we don't need to activate the stress response. The authors list laughter, affection, crying, creative expression, a stress-reducing twenty-second hug, and positive social interactions as other evidence-based actions that complete the stress cycle response.

Our menstrual cycle tends to tell us how we're managing stress. Under high levels of acute or chronic stress, we might experience more PMS symptoms, increased pain and cramping during our periods, irregular cycles, or struggles with infertility. This doesn't have to be our story. Completing the stress cycle doesn't eliminate stress from our lives, but it does give us a way to cope and helps prevent stress from slowly, painfully killing us. Then, we can start working on the source of that stress and making incremental changes to the root cause of our burnout or dysregulated cortisol levels. Our menstruating years challenge us to pause, rest, breathe, and then decide that the story of these incredible years should not solely revolve around stress about jobs, children, painful periods, or anything else. These years are a time to resist cultural norms that perpetuate the unpaid work burden and fight back against patriarchal messages that we should always produce and always take care of others before we care for ourselves. The reproductive years are an opportunity to fully experience our menstruality. These are the years when we study ourselves, transform, and gain a sense of embodied wisdom in which we learn to trust what we need and treat ourselves with deeply compassionate care and attention.

Complete the Stress Cycle

MOVE	Physical activity is the most effective way to complete the stress cycle. We tend to move less during stressful times, which is when we need movement the most. By making movement like daily walking a habit, it's easier to continue to move during periods of heightened stress.
BREATHE	The stress response is quelled by deep breathing. Breathing deep into your belly can slow your heart rate, stabilize or lower blood pressure, and downshift your physiological response to stress.
TEND-AND-BEFRIEND	Research finds that when cisgender women are stressed, they are more cooperative, caring, and compassionate. This is known as the tend-and-befriend response to stress, which reduces fear and increases hope during or after stressful events through the action of seeking social support and spending time communicating with or caring for loved ones. A supportive community is essential, and isolation is especially harmful. Seeking therapy is another way to practice tend-and-befriend theory.
LAUGH	A powerful drug, laughter decreases cortisol and other stress hormones, benefits mental and immune health, alters dopamine and serotonin activity, and improves relationships and overall quality of life.
CRY	Crying in response to physiological stress may help return us to biological homeostasis by regulating heart rate and promoting purposeful breathing.

Self-Care and Movement

Breathe

The autonomic nervous system is composed of the sympathetic (flight/fight/freeze) system (SNS) and the parasympathetic (rest/digest) system (PNS). The vagus nerve—a cranial nerve with broad body-wide effects—modulates the PNS and is regulated by breathing. One of its jobs is to relay relaxing messages from the central nervous system to the body. During inhalation and when our SNS is activated, vagus nerve activity is inhibited whereas exhalation and slow respiration cycles activate the vagus nerve. Two excellent breathing techniques that activate the vagus nerve and shift your body into a rest-and-digest state are diaphragmatic breathing and alternate nostril breathing.

Diaphragmatic Breathing

Sit up straight or lie down with your knees bent and feet firmly planted on the ground, both hip-width apart. Place one hand on your chest and one hand on your belly. Breathe in through your nose and allow the breath to slowly fill your lower belly. Feel the hand on your belly gently rise. Engage your abdominal muscles and exhale all of the air out of your nose. To improve focus and breath control, count to 5 on the inhale, hold for 5 seconds, then exhale for 5 seconds during each round. Repeat for 5 to 10 minutes.

Alternate Nostril Breathing

Sit up straight and bring your right hand up to your face. Place your right thumb on your right nostril. With the right nostril closed, inhale through your left nostril. Using your right index finger close the left nostril, momentarily closing both nostrils, then lift your right thumb, exhaling out the right nostril. (You can also do this with your opposite hand if you prefer, just reverse the directions.) Repeat. Again, try inhaling for 5 seconds, holding for 5 seconds, and exhaling for 5 seconds each round. Continue cycling for 10 to 20 breaths or around 5 minutes.

Find a Walking Buddy

It is well-established through research and day-to-day life experience that social interactions, both the quality and quantity, affect our mental and physical health, behavior, and mortality risk. Our social interactions accumulate over a lifetime and either give us a disadvantage or advantage when it comes to our health. As you might guess, positive social interactions give us a positive health advantage because they come with emotional support and laughter, providing us with a sense of meaning in our life that enhances our mental health. Walking with a friend or partner offers an incredible boost to the quality of life of both walkers. A 2017 paper from *American Psychology* found that walking together supports creativity and a bodily sense of forward progress and also facilitates psychological pathways for conflict resolution. Synchronous movement comes with the benefit of increased empathy and camaraderie. Our postures shift to benefit one another and we experience a sense of shared attention and place in the world.

Free Your Psoas

The psoas is a muscle that lives within our anterior hip joint and lower spine, connecting our upper body to our lower body. It is considered by some to be the most important skeletal muscle in the human body. This complicated and dynamic muscle acts as a stabilizer for the lumbar spine and hips, has a relationship to our nervous system and emotions, and plays a key role in our stress response. Liz Koch, an expert on the psoas, says this bio-intelligent tissue "embodies our deepest urge for survival, and more profoundly, our elemental desire to flourish." Koch says the psoas provides circulatory, emotional, and structural support, and when we regain a "supple, dynamic, and juicy" psoas, we promote healthy organ functioning and reduce stress, which help relieve menstrual cramps. So how can you free your psoas and allow it to flourish? Start with sitting less. Our sitting, stress, and sedentarism abuse our psoas, which longs for movement and play. Here are a few movements to nurture your psoas.

Psoas Resting Position

Start by lying on your back on the floor with your knees bent to 90 degrees, feet flat on the floor, with both knees and feet hip-width apart. Close your eyes and imagine your inhales and exhales moving up and down your spine as you allow your body to relax and sink into the floor. Spend at least 5 minutes in this resting position.

Supported Bridge

Lie on your back in the same position as the resting position, then lift your hips and place a yoga block at the shortest height under your sacrum, making sure it is not under your lower back. Breathe here for 2 to 5 minutes. Remove the block and bring your hips back to the ground. Bring one leg up and, clasping your hands around your knee, pull it toward your shoulder. Allow the other leg to extend straight out and then gently lower it until your heel touches the floor. Hold this stretch for 5 breath cycles on each side.

Chair Differently

My personal favorite Liz Koch movement for unraveling the psoas employs a sturdy chair (no arms and either cushioned or uncushioned), bench, or couch. Start by sitting in the chair, feet planted on the ground, stretching your body, neck, and arms in swaying and circular side-to-side movements. Then, lean your body forward and to the right side, and connect your hands to the ground (spread your fingers so that there is equal distance between each finger and press down evenly on each finger where it meets the palm, creating five points of contact). Shift your weight from your buttocks to your right hip on the chair, placing more weight in your hands, and moving into an inversion as your head hangs down by your hands. In this strong, supported position, start exploring movement with your legs. Reach your left leg up in the air to the side and front, bending the knee and moving slowly, paying attention to sensations in the leg and psoas. Try bending and extending your knees and opening and closing your torso and even reaching one hand forward and back. The purpose of this movement is to find pleasure and fun through exploration. You may feel light and graceful like an upside-down ballet dancer or tight and bound if your muscles are tense. Give yourself time to find a flow and rhythm, 5 minutes or so on each side, and repeat often.

Live by a Daily Rhythm

In some schools, children follow a daily rhythm described as an inhale and exhale. The inhale is the time of day when they concentrate and do projects like drawing, painting, and cooking. During the breathing-in period, kids are usually inside. Each breathing-in period is followed by a breathing-out period, usually outside. The exhale is a time of expansion, exploration, and freedom when kids run and play without structure or direction. The daily rhythm is about balance, and it requires attention and the ability to live in the present moment. Following a similar rhythm as an adult gives us a way to ebb and flow with our changing energy and needs throughout the day. Often, we get caught in a breathing-in period all day with work, caretaking, cleaning, grocery shopping, cooking, eating, responding to messages, and even exercising. Breathe out. The breathing-out period is an essential time of reset, rejuvenation, and rest. Following a work-play-rest rhythm creates calm when there is chaos and quiet moments of stillness when we are too often surrounded by action and noise. Some ways we can breathe out after a long period of inhalation include going outside and moving in nature, napping, meditating, and other quiet, calm, and creative activities.

Nutrition

Nutrition is important during the menstruating years whether or not you decide to become pregnant. That said, the nutrition information in this section is specifically tailored toward fertility (but happens to benefit overall health in people who are and are not trying to conceive). This is because pregnancy, breastfeeding, and caring for a baby are the major energy-intensive events that may occur during the menstruating years. You need a lot of good food to get through these events, otherwise our health—and our babies' health—may suffer. The same foods that build healthy babies also keep your body healthy. A 2018 review published in the *American Journal of Obstetrics and Gynecology* found that folate, vitamin B_{12}, omega-3 fatty acids, and "healthy diets" like the Mediterranean diet (think olive oil, lots of veggies, fish, fruit, and whole grains) had a positive effect on fertility while diets high in trans fats, processed and red meat, sugar, and potatoes appeared to negatively affect fertility. Before you ditch potatoes and move to the Mediterranean, it's important to understand that these studies have limitations and offer a shallow understanding of the complex and layered world of food and how it relates to fertility. Of note, the study didn't examine a few nutrients that are especially important for our reproductive health including choline, iodine, glycine, preformed vitamin A, vitamin K_2, DHA, and zinc.

Choline

Vital to all of the cells in our body and their structural integrity, choline is an essential nutrient that is also needed to produce the neurotransmitter acetylcholine, which is important for mood, brain and nervous system functions, and muscle control. Choline is especially critical during pregnancy and breastfeeding as it affects placental function, neurodevelopment—including attention, self-regulation, vision, and epigenetic programming—including growth, brain development, and chronic disease risk. The current recommended daily requirement for choline is 425 mg/day, 450 mg/day during pregnancy, and 550 mg/day during lactation. According to several studies, these recommendations aren't nearly high enough and find that our choline needs more than double during pregnancy and go up even higher during lactation. The easiest way to increase choline intake is to eat eggs—two egg yolks contain around 250 mg of choline. The best sources are animal proteins, such as beef (especially beef liver), poultry, cod, and dairy products. Cruciferous vegetables like cauliflower and broccoli also contain a small amount of choline. Anywhere from 90 to 95 percent of pregnant people don't consume enough choline, so adding more choline-rich foods and/or supplementing with choline during pregnancy is especially important.

Iodine

A 2018 study in *Human Reproduction* found that cisgender women who had moderate to severe iodine deficiency took longer to become pregnant compared to the iodine sufficient group. This study is important because while research has long identified that iodine deficiency is a common problem worldwide, the relationship between iodine deficiency and reproductive health hasn't received much attention. The greatest impact iodine deficiency has is on thyroid function. Simply, if there isn't enough iodine, the thyroid can't make enough hormones, and this leads to hypothyroidism, which is linked to neurodevelopmental problems in a fetus, miscarriage, postpartum thyroiditis, and infertility. The best food sources of iodine include fish like cod and tuna, seaweeds, shrimp, other seafood, and eggs and dairy products.

Skip Sugar

Eating too much sugar in the form of sweets, sugary drinks, and refined carbohydrates has a negative effect on fertility and disrupts hormonal health, leading to conditions like insulin resistance, which is associated with PCOS. Excess sugar consumption leads to many body-wide issues including disrupted satiety signaling, increased stress, fatigue, and increased body fat. Sugar is remarkably addictive because it overstimulates reward systems in the brain, which leads to intense sugar cravings. The chronic overactivation of what is called the "food reward" response harms brain health. Studies find that diets high in sugar are bad for memory, mood, learning skills, and increase brain inflammation, which is linked to anxiety and depression. Most people consume more than 22 teaspoons of sugar daily (kids consume even more at 34 teaspoons a day). This is significantly more than the American Heart Association recommendation, which suggests limiting added sugar to 6 teaspoons daily for women and 9 teaspoons for men. Because sugar is so delicious, and so hard to stop eating, but so important to reduce to improve overall health, taking a multi-faceted approach to breaking the sugar habit is often required.

Here are some suggestions for managing sugar cravings and reducing sugar intake:

- Get the sugary drinks, cookies, candies, and other high-sugar food out of your house so they aren't there to tempt you.

- Read labels when buying new products. Food manufacturers slip sugar into many foods, especially drinks and products labeled "low fat." Look for food with zero added sugars.

- Add more nutrient-dense food to your diet such as fruits, vegetables, protein, healthy fat, whole grains, and nut and seed butters. These foods help stabilize blood sugar levels, which reduces blood sugar crashes followed by sugar cravings.

- Retrain your taste buds. Eat plain yogurt, sweet potatoes, caramelized onions, squash, fruit, and other naturally sweet foods while eliminating sugary treats. Your taste buds will recalibrate. Bitter foods such as watercress and arugula and fermented and sour foods also help reset your taste buds so you crave less sugar.

- Do a sugar detox. For some people, gradually eating less sugar works best, but for others, the best approach to decreasing sugar intake is to quit all added sugar intake for something like thirty days.

- Manage your stress, move more, and get enough sleep. All of these actions help reduce sugar cravings.

The Menopausal
Transition

AGE ±40–60

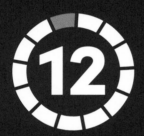

When most of us think about menopause, we think of symptoms: hot flashes, irritability, irregular cycles, lack of libido, vaginal dryness, weight gain, depression, anxiety, more hair on your chin and less on your head. We think of loss—loss of memory, loss of sexual desire, and loss of our partners to younger, sexier women. We're taught to think of menopause as a pathological period of hormone deficiency that catapults us out of our fertile years and into the ether of old age and unimportance. This chapter isn't about minimizing or denying the symptoms that may accompany the menopausal transition. It is about changing the way we think about menopause and doing our best to prepare for this transition.

Menopause is defined as the one-year anniversary of your last menstrual period. The menopausal transition, on the other hand, can last for years as our ovarian hormone levels decrease and we are spurred on a physiological, emotional, and spiritual journey. How we navigate through the end of the menstruating years reflects how well we've taken care of ourselves up to that point and how well we're able to listen to our body and give it what it needs. Our menstruating years are like training wheels for the menopausal transition. We first learn how to pay attention to our cycles so that we may know ourselves and our bodies more deeply. We learn about how self-care, movement, and healthy food contribute to our overall well-being. Our transition out of our fertile years is the test. Did we address and reduce chronic stress and stressors? Did we make space for ourselves to navigate changes in our energy? Did we cultivate a team of allies and relationships that support us with respect as we walk through these years?

Many people haven't spent time contemplating the lived experience of menopause, so the idea of preparing for menopause might feel foreign. Despite the large cultural silence and inattention surrounding this phase, we can expect to live a third, or even half, of our lives in our postmenopausal years. The way we approach this next season deeply affects how we experience it. Studies show that people who expect the menopausal transition to be difficult experience more menopause symptoms and higher levels of depression. Higher levels of depression during menopause come with a twofold higher risk of cognitive impairment and dementia later in life. In her book *The Slow Moon Climbs*, Susan P. Mattern writes that the way we experience menopause is largely, but not entirely, dependent on what our beliefs and expectations are. Western European medicine has popularized the perception of menopause as a dangerous condition of estrogen deficiency since the 1700s. This "fundamentally wrong view of menopause," Mattern writes, is expanding its reach, globally influencing the cultural perceptions and experience of menopause. Just like we're taught to expect pain and bad moods before our first period, we learn that menopause is another feminine curse we must suffer through in silence.

Nothing could be further from the truth. One of the key steps we must take in preparing for menopause is a fierce and dedicated resistance to negative stereotypes and pathological descriptions of this phase. We do change, it isn't always easy, but this change is normal. Another key step is education. Whether this transition is just around the corner or decades in the future, there is no time like the present to gain understanding; each lifestyle suggestion and adaptation in this chapter, while geared toward the menopausal transition, also promotes overall health at any age and life stage. This chapter will explore the science and lived experience of menopause so we know what to expect and how to prepare for this shift. We'll examine the neurological basis of menopausal symptoms and how to take better care of our brains in the years leading up to and during the menopausal transition, which reduces symptoms *and* reduces Alzheimer's risk. My hope is that, after reading this primer on the menopausal transition, you'll view menopause not as a dreadful end where we shrivel up and have nothing left to offer, but as an essential, normal, and valuable transition to a rich season of life.

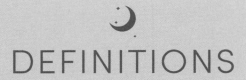

DEFINITIONS

PREMENOPAUSE/THE MENSTRUATING YEARS: When we're still experiencing normal menstrual cycles. Some people start to feel a shift in their energy and self-concept before they experience changes in their menstrual cycle, usually in their late thirties or early forties.

PERIMENOPAUSE: The years leading up to menopause, usually starting in our late forties (but can start in our thirties), marked by changes in our cycle such as a shortened follicular phase, anovulatory cycles, skipped cycles, or lighter or heavier flows.

THE MENOPAUSAL TRANSITION: Progressive hormone changes that transition us from the menstruating years, when menstrual cycles are regular, ovulatory, and predictable, to the final menstrual period.

MENOPAUSE: When we stop having menstrual periods for twelve consecutive months, we've officially gone through menopause. Huge variability in age exists, but the average age to experience menopause is fifty-one. The age of menopause is affected by your mother's age at menopause, BMI, tobacco and alcohol use, and other factors. Menopause happens to nonbinary, cis women, trans men, and intersex people.

- **PREMATURE MENOPAUSE:** Menses ends before age 40

- **EARLY MENOPAUSE:** Age 50–59

- **LATE MENOPAUSE:** Age 60+

- **SURGICAL MENOPAUSE:** Surgical removal of both ovaries

- **MEDICAL MENOPAUSE:** Permanent damage to both ovaries following chemotherapy or radiation. People using gender-affirming hormones including testosterone and estrogen blockers may experience menopause-like symptoms when either discontinuing hormones (say, for a surgery) or restarting the hormones.

POSTMENOPAUSE: On day 366, after 365 days of no menstrual cycle (or after surgical ovarian removal), we're postmenopausal. Following menopause, we're in our postmenopausal years. In general, symptoms experienced during the menopausal transition decrease during this time.

Menopause on the Brain

Before we're officially labeled perimenopausal, many people are conscious of an internal shift and experience emotional fragility, loss of sleep, anxiety, or a sense of just not feeling like themselves during their late reproductive years when they are still normally cycling. Some feel these changes start as early as their late thirties while others feel them in their early or midforties.

During the early transition, our menstrual cycles are mostly intact, following the rhythm we've learned to track and understand over the years. The late transition comes with greater cycle irregularity with periods disappearing for months at a time, showing back up, and disappearing again until they are gone for good. These transitions have been further broken down into stages detailing the specific hormone shifts, the first of which is often a rise in follicle stimulating hormone (FSH). This increase in FSH signals our remaining follicles to more rapidly grow and develop, which shortens the follicular phase of the menstrual cycle and contributes to the irregular menstrual cycles that characterize perimenopause.

Around age thirty-five, we start producing more variable levels of progesterone from month to month. During perimenopause, our production of progesterone starts to decline and estrogen secretion may become more erratic. Because estrogen and progesterone are interrelated and affect each other's levels, less progesterone production can result in increased estrogen production. Progesterone is our sleep-promoting and soothing hormone, so when it's low and our progesterone and estrogen levels change, we may experience symptoms such insomnia, anxiety, irritability, painful periods, and heightened anger, or what some going through this transition call "perimenopausal rage." Even though our periods become irregular, we may still ovulate or we may not ovulate but have high or low

Hormones and Menstruation throughout Life

	MENARCHE (AVG. AGE 12)	MENSTRUATING YEARS		
		Early	Peak	Late (late 30s–40s)
HORMONES		Normal FSH		↑FSH, erratic estrogen, ↓progesterone
MENSTRUAL CYCLE		Variable to regular	Regular	
DURATION OF STAGE		Avg. span age 12–51		

estrogen levels (meaning effective contraception methods are still needed). This time of irregularity and unpredictability is known as the speed bump of the menopausal transition, but it's more like a bumpy dirt road where one minute we're driving along smoothly, and the next, we're getting jostled and rocked uncomfortably, and then the road is smooth again, then bumpy again. This bumpy time is when we're more likely to experience the symptoms we commonly associate with menopause such as hot flashes, poor sleep, and mood disturbances.

These symptoms vary widely based on age, race, ethnicity, lifestyle, and genetics. Hot flashes, the cardinal feature of menopause, vary in length and severity, with some people experiencing them for years and others barely at all. What's important to understand about these symptoms, according to the neuroscientist Lisa Mosconi, is that they originate in the brain. That is, they are neurological symptoms first. Hot flashes, for example, happen because our brain isn't adequately regulating our body temperature.

MENOPAUSAL TRANSITION (AVG. AGE 47)		MENOPAUSE (AVG. AGE 51)	POSTMENOPAUSE	
Early	Late	1 year no cycles	Early	Late
↑FSH, ↓estrogen, ↓progesterone			↑FSH, ↓estrogen, ↓progesterone	
Variable (>7 days different from normal)	Skipped cycles + 60 days with no period		None	
Highly variable, avg. length transition 4 years Early onset associated w/longer transition			4 years	Until death

Our sex hormones are involved in brain function and influence brain connectivity. Estrogen, for example, is key for energy production in the brain and maintaining homeostasis. It protects our brain cells, keeping them active and healthy, and supports neurological functions such as memory, attention, and planning.

You can probably see where this is going, and yes, menopause has a huge impact on our brains. Through her research, Mosconi has found that some women in the menopausal transition show an increased accumulation of amyloid plaques, a major red flag for Alzheimer's disease. What researchers know about Alzheimer's is that brain changes often happen decades before the onset of symptoms. Mosconi and other scientists find that the transition to menopause is a risky time for our brains. We lose some of the neuroprotective benefits of estrogen, and our brains must adjust to this new hormonal landscape. It is during this adjustment period that we're most vulnerable and experience issues with memory, forgetfulness, mood swings, anxiety, and depression. We're also more susceptible to diabetes, obesity, and heart disease, which can further affect brain health. This time of heightened neural vulnerability, Mosconi says, is often when health risks turn into full-fledged medical issues.

This all sounds like very bad, doomsday news, especially since cisgender women experience brain diseases like Alzheimer's at much higher rates than cisgender men. But one quote from Mosconi illustrates the complexity of this time period well:

> Your genetics—your age, your gender, and your family—form the hand you've been dealt. But winning and losing have less to do with those cards than with the way you play the game: your environment, lifestyle, medical history, and, especially for women, hormonal health.

Her work, while zoomed in on the science of the brain, is heavily focused on prevention. She says that taking better care of our brains during our reproductive years and through the menopausal transition dramatically reduces Alzheimer's risk and can decrease the severity of menopause symptoms. Some of the major evidence-based ways to take care of our brains involve eating a healthy diet full of anti-inflammatory foods (the Mediterranean diet is backed by the most research), moving often, engaging in consistent and conscientious intellectual and social activities (think Scrabble with friends), practicing stress management and reduction, getting restful sleep, nurturing hormonal health, and avoiding environmental toxins and behaviors like smoking.

Our late reproductive and perimenopausal years are the time to be ambitious about protecting our health and preventing dementia later in life. We tend to think of conditions like Alzheimer's as genetic diseases, but more and more research is finding that our genes are only one part of our health story. Our health is multigenic, meaning we have multiple genes that interact and influence our well-being and longevity. Crucially, Mosconi points out that, in general, there aren't single "bad" genes, just genes that come with a higher risk of making us sick, and we can modify that risk with our lifestyle choices.

The following section on the lived experience of the menopausal transition presents one representation of how you *might* feel during this phase that highlights common menopausal themes and is rooted in Western social structure and patterning. But it is by no means the only possibility; an important part of your menopausal education is following your own path.

A Long Fall

Alexandra Pope, an educator who teaches people about the lived experience of the menstrual cycle and menopause, describes the menopausal transition as a long fall preceding a deep winter that then blossoms into a second spring or summer, aka the postmenopausal years. Perimenopause is similar to the fall season of the luteal phase, specifically the late luteal phase, when we may experience PMS symptoms. This autumnal season, however, is more profound than the luteal phase. It is a time of great physical, emotional, and spiritual change when we rethink and reevaluate everything in our lives and explore a new world within ourselves.

The menopausal transition is often described as a hole we fall into or a gap in time when everything that we thought we knew, everything that used to make sense, just doesn't make sense anymore. It's a time when we're deeply tired and feel compelled to retreat, to get away from responsibility and the normal pressures and demands of our lives. "Deep inside, you kind of want to walk out the door and say there's food in the freezer," Pope says, "I'll be back when I'm back."

In this time of vulnerability, the most crucial step we can take is to slow down. When we try to continue at the same rate at work and at home, if we sacrifice sleep, a healthy diet, or self-care, we pay the price with more physical symptoms. When we try to avoid, ignore, or power through these physical symptoms, they become worse and we might feel embarrassed, deeply uncomfortable, and ashamed of our bodies; like they are betraying us. This can bring up deep anxiety and a sense of panic. When we don't nurture ourselves with what Pope calls "fierce self-care practices," we risk spiraling through the menopausal transition with misery and reduced emotional and physical resilience.

What we need is agency and space to take care of ourselves. We need to cultivate an environment of safety, respect, and inclusivity for us and those around us to understand that we're going through something real and transformational. Menopause changes us and whoever is around us, and this is the time when we need our partners to step up and help lessen the care burden we often acutely face during these years. Slowing down means becoming more aware of how we use our time and energy because our tolerance for stress is both physically and emotionally lower. Pope adds that it's critical during this time to address any grief we feel, especially the grief that may arrive if we didn't have children but wanted to. Depending on our health, we're likely to negotiate the most extreme physical symptoms of menopause such as hot flashes, sleep problems, and fatigue for six to twelve months. It is during this time of disturbance that we tend to feel overwhelmed and want everything in our lives to stop for a little while.

There are compelling reasons to nurture our health during the menopausal transition. As discussed earlier, taking care of ourselves helps keep our brains healthy, which decreases the chances that we'll develop dementia and reduces the severity of menopause symptoms. Additionally, on the other side of this menopausal speed bump, our postmenopausal years are waiting for us. We have an opportunity to step into these years with a renewed sense of power and a deep sense of who we are and what matters to us.

So far, we've looked at how our experience of menopause is largely dependent on our expectations and beliefs and that during the late reproductive years through menopause hormone production becomes more erratic, leading to irregular periods, frequent anovulatory cycles, and other symptoms before we finally menstruate for the last time. The transition from one life stage to the next is both a physiological and psychospiritual journey, a serious and real disturbance of self from which we come out changed into the next version of ourselves.

We can deepen our understanding of how we experience menopause, and what we might do to improve our experience, by expanding our understanding of how our brains work. The revolutionary psychologist and neuroscientist Lisa Feldman Barrett explains that our brains run our bodies using something akin to a budget, meaning we have certain resources—nutrients, water, electrolytes, and hormones—and our brain's job is to make economic decisions about where to put them. Actions such as running and sweating withdraw from that budget while sleeping and eating act as deposits. These actions are meant to keep us alive. "Your brain didn't evolve for you to see and think and feel," Barrett says, "it evolved to regulate your body." To accomplish this immense task, the brain is constantly guessing what our body needs. Past experiences combined with input from our environment and physical sensations are the ingredients the brain uses to guess how we should feel.

Most of the processes the brain regulates can't be felt, but we can feel mood. "Your mood is like a barometer for the health of your body," Barrett writes. "It's with you every moment of your life, though much of the time it's in the background and you don't notice it." Our brain doesn't separately budget for mental versus physical functions because the distinction between the mind and body is meaningless for the brain. In a 2020 article in the *New York Times*, Barrett wrote,

> Anxiety does not cause stomach aches; rather, feelings of anxiety and stomach aches are both ways that human brains make sense of physical discomfort. There is no such thing as a purely mental cause because every mental experience has roots in the physical budgeting of your body. This is one reason physical actions like taking a deep breath, or getting more sleep, can be surprisingly helpful in addressing problems we traditionally view as psychological.

Applying Barrett's body-budget metaphor, we can see how the menopausal transition stresses our body budget and how some of our symptoms may be rooted in how the brain is guessing we should feel based on the ingredients it has access to. If our ingredients are reinforcing negative predictions about the experience of menopause and we've overdrawn our budget (easy to do in a culture that doesn't value sleep, healthy food, or rest), our health is more likely to suffer.

Budgeting well requires a certain kind of literacy. In the case of finances, we need financial literacy; for the body, we need body literacy. Part of that literacy involves improving our emotional intelligence, which requires actual literacy. "Words seed your concepts," Barrett writes, "concepts drive your predictions, predictions regulate your body budget (which is how your brain anticipates and fulfills your body's energy needs), and your body budget determines how you feel." Expanding our emotional vocabulary from the limited and binary (for example, sad versus happy) to a more descriptive and nuanced range improves what is called our "emotional granularity." So, instead of sad, consider the nuances of: inconsolable, woeful, despondent, regretful, miserable, melancholic, or gloomy, and instead of happy, try: content, merry, lighthearted, ecstatic, euphoric, or delighted. Research shows that people with higher emotional granularity use less medication, go to the doctor less, are hospitalized less, and are more flexible when regulating their emotions. In other words, they are much healthier, just from their expanded use of words!

The other lesson I want to highlight from Barrett (though there are many more you can find in her book *How Emotions Are Made: The Secret Life of the Brain*) is the value of emotional deconstruction and recategorization.

Emotional Granularity

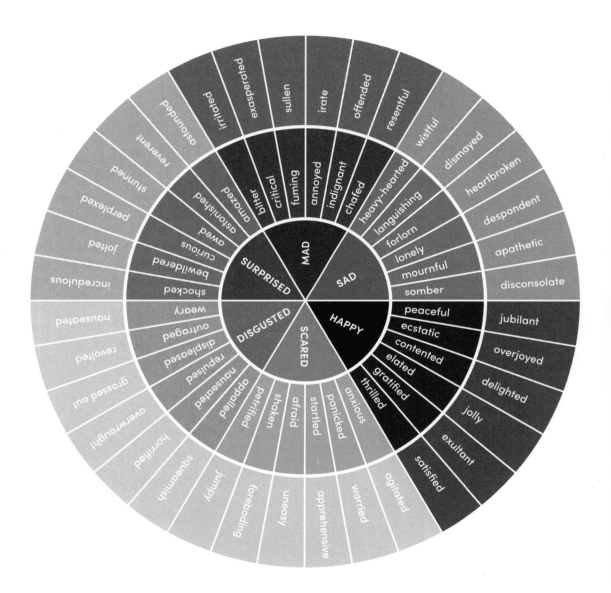

exploring the four seasons of life

For example, if you deconstruct anxiety or fear down to their physical sensations—a racing heartbeat—and then recategorize a racing heartbeat as a natural coping strategy, it helps separate a negative emotion from a physical sensation. What this practice does is change how we interpret our physical state. "Learn to deconstruct a feeling into its mere physical sensations," Barrett writes, "rather than letting those sensations be a filter through which you view the world."

Let's look at how we might deconstruct and recategorize a physical sensation like hot flashes. Say we feel a hot flash and our brains construct a feeling of panic and anxiety. By deconstructing these feelings back to the hot flash, then recategorizing them as a normal part of the menopausal transition, we may then take a deep breath, drink some water, close our eyes and breathe, go for a walk outside, or find a supportive group or provider to help us. These actions don't eliminate the physical sensation, but they do provide us with coping mechanisms and change how we interpret menopausal symptoms. We're not losing our minds; our bodies are changing, and we need to take care of them with greater attention and care.

Can you see how powerful and important it is for our health and well-being to expand our vocabulary of menopause and recategorize our experience of the menopausal transition? It's the difference between blindly accepting that we're doomed versus asking, "What can I do to make this experience different and better?" We can ask body-budgeting questions that slow us down and put us in tune with our bodies like, "Did I drink enough water today? Do I need to spend time with friends? Did I get enough sleep last night?" We can also change our ingredients by doing things such as taking a deep breath, changing our environment, and creating new experiences that change our brain's prediction patterns and thus how we feel.

I didn't realize that when I dove into the books, research, stories, and cultural traditions surrounding menopause and the menopausal transition that I would start my own journey of emotional recategorization. Slowly, my worries about the end of my fertility and the accompanying symptoms were recategorized into a patient kind of anticipation for this next phase, which is the exact opposite of how our culture teaches us to feel about menopause. I also didn't realize that increasing my understanding of the menopausal transition with vocabulary like "normal," "biological," "healthy," and "transformation" would provide me with greater emotional granularity, or more ways to think about menopause via stories and language. By reframing this experience and learning more words to describe it, we might just change our entire lived experience of this transformation.

Self-Care and Movement

Band Together

The physiological symptoms of menopause are just one part, and potentially not even the most important part, of going through the menopausal transition. A 2019 paper found that menopause is a social experience as much as it is a biological one. Descriptions and stories of shame, isolation, transformation, and even hilarity shared between people experiencing this transition provide meaning and context to their experience. We are a social species, and we regulate one another's body budgets. This means that the company we keep and the exchanges we make influence our physical health and our nervous system. Studies find that people with more support and resilience experience fewer menopausal symptoms. During this time of transition, it is important to find social connections with those who are going through similar experiences or who are knowledgeable about all aspects of the menopausal transition. This can come from both in-person relationships or supportive forums, websites, and groups. Some people also greatly benefit from menopause health coaching, which among other improvements in general health, has been shown to improve quality of life and reduce depression and the severity of symptoms.

Have a Midlife Movement Crisis

During the menopausal transition, some people experience weight gain and body composition changes such as increased belly fat. We might also find ourselves falling into more sedentary habits like sitting more, especially if we're fatigued from sleep disturbances and mood changes. When we feel stagnation, especially the sedentary kind, instead of swapping our Subaru for a Maserati, we might instead consider transforming our environment in a way that forces us to move more. You could sit on the floor instead of in chairs, hang monkey bars in your house or backyard, walk to nearby places for errands, or plant and tend to a garden (all of which increase your mobility, strength, aerobic capacity, and muscle mass).

We often need much more rest during this phase too, so cleaning up your sleep hygiene (see page 161), taking a nap, or meditating every day helps keep our body budget from bankrupting. Think of your fitness—your muscle mass, strength, mobility, and aerobic capacity—as some of the most important tools you carry with you into your postmenopausal years that protect you from age-related degeneration. Hone these tools by performing diverse movements such as hiking, walking, hanging, and squatting, and incorporate high-intensity movements like lifting and jumping. If you're finding yourself sitting more, remember that changing your environment changes your brain, which affects your mood and behavior.

Cultivate Gratitude and Reciprocity

In her 2020 essay "The Serviceberry," Robin Wall Kimmerer writes that when we think of food like the serviceberry not as a commodity or product but as a gift, our intuitive response is gratitude to all of the elements—the rain, sun, soil, other plants, and people—that cultivated and led us to this gift. Gratitude, she writes, "is the thread that connects us in a deep relationship, simultaneously physical and spiritual, as our bodies are fed and spirits are nourished by the sense of belonging, which is the most vital of foods." Gratitude cultivates a feeling of abundance and generates the next response: reciprocity. What can we do to show the plants and our shared environment that we are grateful for their generosity? We could water the plants, share them with our neighbors, plant more, donate to environmental organizations—the list goes on. Why is this so important, especially during the menopausal transition? Patriarchal and consumerist culture doesn't acknowledge bodily rites of passage like menopause, so it is up to us to strongly make a place for ourselves in the world. "To name the world as a gift is to feel one's membership in the web of reciprocity," Kimmerer writes. "It makes you happy—and it makes you accountable." If we see our earth, ourselves, and our relationship to the earth as a gift, we're more likely to take care of the whole.

Go Off the Grid

Sleep problems, insomnia, and fatigue are some of the most challenging symptoms associated with the menopausal transition. But there is a way to rapidly reset your circadian rhythm, improve sleep, and reduce stress and depression: wilderness camping. Spending time in nature is necessary for our health. Time spent outside in nature, whether in the park closest to your home or in the wild backcountry, reduces blood pressure and lowers stress hormone levels while giving us a sense of clarity and awe.

A 2017 study from *Current Biology* found that camping in nature realigns our circadian rhythm to a natural light-dark cycle. In two different studies, the researchers measured a group of people's melatonin levels in a lab, equipped them with wearable devices that measured their sleep time, and then sent them off into the woods for a weeklong camping trip. One group was studied on a summer camping trip and the other on a winter camping trip. The researchers found that before going on their camping trip, people's internal clocks were delayed by around 2.5 hours. A delay in circadian timing is associated with a whole host of health problems such as diabetes, obesity, and substance abuse along with daytime sleepiness and negative cognitive performance. Both the summer and winter campers were exposed to much higher levels of natural light and sleep time occurred 2.5 hours earlier and lasted, on average, 2.3 hours longer. Their melatonin rhythms adjusted to match the environment—shortening during the summer when there is more natural light and lengthening in the winter when there is less. The researchers also looked at the effects of camping during the weekend. When people are at home, they tend to stay up later and sleep in, which causes enhanced delays to their circadian rhythms. But, after a two-day camping trip, campers' internal clocks shifted earlier. Spending just two nights in the wilderness rapidly resets our circadian timing: we sleep better, move more, and our bodies adapt to the solar rhythm of our environment.

Nutrition

A common thread that runs through the menopausal transition is a realization that we can't "get away" with eating sugar, processed foods, and refined carbohydrates. These foods cause spikes in blood sugar, and research shows that people with imbalanced blood sugar and insulin resistance experience hot flashes, night sweats, and other menopausal symptoms more often. Visceral fat, also known as intra-abdominal fat, is associated with insulin resistance and linked to metabolic disturbances that increase our risk of developing breast cancer, cardiovascular disease, and type 2 diabetes. Food—what we eat, how we eat, and how much—is so important during this phase because it has a huge impact on how we experience our symptoms *and* our risk of developing chronic diseases.

Stabilize Blood Sugar Levels

Step one to balancing your blood sugar levels is to reduce or eliminate your intake of refined carbohydrates (like white flour), foods with added and refined sugar (juice, soda, sauces, muffins, cookies), and processed foods (fast food, chips, sweets). Step two is to eat more of the type of foods that contribute to glucose stability such as fish, chicken, grass-fed meats, tempeh, and beans along with plenty of vegetables and healthy fats such as olive oil, avocado, nuts, and seeds. Step three is to add herbs like cinnamon, garlic, ginger, oregano, turmeric, basil, cumin, and chili, which help boost flavor and improve blood sugar stability. Step four: get rid of the artificial sweeteners that disturb your gut microbes. Step five: move your body often and in different ways every day. And step six, prioritize sleep. All of these steps overlap and lead to improved energy and balanced blood sugar levels.

Eat Calm

A 2019 study from *Cell Metabolism* found that stressed mice became obese more quickly than non-stressed mice eating the same high-calorie food. Under stress, the researchers found that a specific molecule in the amygdala called neuropeptide Y (NPY) was over-activated and led to a change in the mice's response to food and stress, increasing food intake, insulin levels, and obesity. Under chronic stress, blood insulin levels were slightly elevated, but in combination with a high-calorie diet, insulin levels were ten times higher than mice in the stress-free environment. We need more research on stress-induced obesity in humans, but animal studies like this one give us insight into how stress may affect our metabolism.

Based on this and other research, setting an intention to reduce stress before meals and eat mindfully may improve metabolism.

Here are some ideas for reducing stress before and during mealtime:

- Close your eyes, take a deep breath, and either vocally or silently express gratitude or a prayer for the food you're about to eat.

- Eat without distractions such as phones or television and with good company when possible.

- Eat outside in nature or even next to a tree with a pretty view.

- Listen to soothing music while eating.

- Start your meal with a mindful bite while you thoroughly smell, taste, chew, and enjoy the experience of eating.

Stick with the Basics

When you're going through the menopausal transition, certain targeted nutrition advice will probably find you. These include but are not limited to: being told you need to balance, reset, or detox your hormones; eat a ketogenic diet or practice intermittent fasting or other restrictive dieting; and/or take supplements. While some of these approaches work for some people, they aren't for everyone. What matters during this transition, and over a lifetime, is supporting our ability to consistently choose that which sustains and maintains our health. These basics can be simplified into the core themes of this book: eating diverse, nutrient-dense food; moving your body often and in different ways; resting and sleeping enough; hydrating; and nurturing your mental health. Though we know these basics, there is often a disconnect between knowing and doing. We can narrow this space by improving our self-awareness and understanding that taking care of ourselves is a lifelong journey that is characterized not by perfection and restriction but by compassion and resilience.

The Postmenopausal Years

AGE 51–THE END

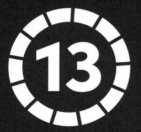

13

Orca whale grandmothers are havens for ecological knowledge—such as how to survive when salmon supply is low—and they become natural leaders during their post-reproductive years, developing closer ties to infant whales through protection and support. When an orca grandmother dies, her whale grandchildren face a reduced survival rate in the two years following her death.

Very few mammals go through the menopausal transition and go on to live long post-reproductive lives, but humans and some whales do, and a suspected reason we live long past our fertile years may be because grandmothers help raise their grandchildren and improve their chance of survival. This theory, called the grandmother hypothesis, was first proposed in the 1960s. That grandmas improve the chances that their grandchildren will survive makes sense in an instinctual way, but beyond being a nice idea, this theory is supported by strong data and mathematical models, which are commonly used by evolutionary biologists to demonstrate what might have happened with our human ancestors a few million years ago. Kristen Hawkes, a distinguished professor of anthropology at the University of Utah, is one of the primary researchers responsible for the robust data in support of this theory. In the 1980s, while studying the Aché hunter-gatherers in Eastern Paraguay and Hadza foragers in Tanzania, she observed that the older women were incredibly productive and hardworking. They were very successful foragers, and their productivity allowed younger women to have a new baby before their previous child could forage well enough to feed itself. In these traditional hunter-gatherer societies, young children and mothers with small babies still participated in foraging, but Hawkes and her colleagues found that the health of the older, weaned child largely depended on how much food their grandmother could forage and share with them. Because of this survival benefit, the evolutionary theory goes that natural selection favored longer postmenopausal lifespans that allowed us to live much longer than our primate cousins.

Intuitive as it might seem, this theory is actually pretty progressive as an evolutionary idea. As discussed in chapter one, our two main evolutionary drives are reproduction and survival. In evolutionary theory, this tends to imply that we only have value during our fertile years. The grandmother hypothesis flips this thinking on its head because it shows that we have reproductive and survival value across our lifespans—first as mothers keeping our babies alive, then as grandparents helping to keep our grandchildren alive. Further, it explains our species' unique longevity. Hawkes says our evolution and lineage favored post-fertile women because of "the contribution they were making to the ancestry of future generations."

As important as the grandmother hypothesis suggests that our postmenopausal years are to the survival of children and the longevity of our species, the treatment of and attitude toward those who are postmenopausal is disappointing both presently and historically. Around the same time that scientists started isolating hormones and learning more about the endocrine system in the 1920s and 1930s, some doctors and pharmaceutical companies started calling menopause a "hormone deficiency disease." Like a person with diabetes who needed insulin, the claim was that menopausal women needed hormones, specifically estrogen. Menopause was reframed as pathological instead of a natural part of growing older. As a capitalistic and patriarchal culture must, the medicalization of menopause was quickly monetized, predominately by men. In 1966, the gynecologist Robert Wilson wrote the bestselling book *Feminine Forever* wherein he refers to menopause as "castration"—a syndrome that deprives women of their sexual functions. "It makes no difference whether castration is brought about by removing the ovaries with a knife as in their surgical removal—or whether the ovaries shrivel up and die as the result of menopause." he wrote, "In either case, the effect is the same: the woman becomes the equivalent of a eunuch."

Wilson—of course—had an answer to the "hormone deficiency disease" of menopause: just take estrogen. He asserted that estrogen therapy would not only save women from their shriveling genitals but it would also restore their youth, balance their bodies, and allow them to remain "feminine forever." Like the elixir vitae made up of mashed animal testicles that ancient alchemists prescribed to cure all sorts of ailments and reverse aging (see page 12), Wilson made a similar promise that estrogen therapy would reverse the ill effects of menopause and allow women to age gradually and gracefully—and "normally," like a healthy male. Perhaps unsurprising now, but scandalous then, it was discovered after Wilson's death that the book was funded entirely by one of the biggest manufacturers of estrogen therapy, the pharmaceutical company Wyeth-Ayerst.

In the 1970s, studies found that high levels of unopposed estrogen supplementation were associated with an increased risk of endometrial cancer, but researchers found that lowering the dose of estrogen and combining it with progesterone reduced endometrial cancer risk. Recall that estrogen increases the thickness of the endometrium, while progesterone limits this thickening effect, so if you only have estrogen acting on the endometrium, the tissue volume increases (endometrial hyperplasia) and may progress to endometrial cancer. Postmenopausal women who've had a hysterectomy, and therefore don't have endometrial tissue to thicken, can safely take estrogen-only hormone therapy, while those who still have a uterus require the balancing effects of progesterone during treatment. In the late 1980s, hormone replacement therapy was prescribed as a preventative therapy for chronic diseases, but then a study found that coronary events— such as heart attacks and death from heart disease—increased with the use of hormone replacement therapy (HRT). In 2002, a huge study called the Women's Health Initiative (WHI) found that HRT was associated with an increased incidence of coronary heart disease and breast cancer while also *reducing* fractures from osteoporosis and colorectal cancer. Based on these results, the risks appeared to outweigh the benefits of HRT and the trial was prematurely discontinued. Seemingly overnight, HRT users panicked, many doctors stopped prescribing this therapy, and the use of HRT dropped by 46 percent in the United States.

The WHI study had one major problem: it didn't include age stratification, a distinction between outcomes and age. Subsequent analyses show that HRT use in early postmenopausal and younger women (age 50–59) is associated with a reduced risk of heart disease and all-cause mortality when taken in the ten years following menopause. This time period is often referred to as a "window of opportunity," when the benefits of HRT may exceed the risks. Most providers prescribe low dose HRT as short-term therapy for severe symptoms; reevaluation and tapering of hormone therapy is recommended after three to five years of treatment; however, there are no specific time limits on the use of HRT and it is a therapeutic option for people because it alleviates many menopausal symptoms.

When it comes to HRT and other treatments for symptoms related to menopause, an individualized approach is essential. What works for one person may not work for another. Some of us will experience intense hot flashes that majorly interfere with sleep and quality of life, and others will experience minimal symptoms. Apart from calling postmenopausal women "eunuchs" and working in the back pocket of a major pharmaceutical company, Wilson's other big problem was generalizing all women as suffering from a disease of estrogen deficiency. Of this problem, Susan P. Mattern writes,

> To speak of estrogen deficiency is to say that women past menopause do not have as much estrogen as they ideally should; in this view women of reproductive age set the standard for the "right" amount of estrogen. If we assumed that women past menopause had the right amount of estrogen for post-reproductive life, we would not say that they had an estrogen deficiency—just as we do not say that an eight-year-old girl is deficient in estrogen.

Perhaps the bigger issue is our cultural story about the place for women in the world once our ability to reproduce ends. Images that are bound to pop up when you google "postmenopausal" are women with their hands on their foreheads, eyes closed, and misery lining their faces. This image is one of grief and loss, and we are taught that our postmenopausal years are the time we lose our health, youth, sex appeal, emotional control, and societal value. This messaging has the capacity to amplify our fear and anxiety, which can then intensify the severity of the menopausal symptoms we experience. Fortunately, there are better stories to guide us and the way we think about our post-fertile years.

In the nineteenth century, before menopause was pathologized, physicians often described the menopausal transition as a crisis period that women emerged from healthy and strong instead of deficient and weak. In some (not all) cultures, the postmenopausal years are viewed as a season of calmness and freedom from reproductive pressure when postmenopausal individuals' wisdom is valued. Mattern highlights the !Kung foragers, pointing out that "women enjoy peak authority and well-being from the time they become grandmothers or mothers-in-law until they begin to become frail in old age." While writing *The Slow Moon Climbs*, Mattern found that younger people who hadn't yet experienced the end of their fertility were much more negative about this transition into the next life stage than those who had already been through it. It's kind of like, during our reproductive years, we see menopause as a bridge into old age and irrelevance while people on the other side of that bridge are having a picnic in the sunshine.

VULVAS AND VAGINAS

The term *genitourinary* refers to the genital and urinary system and structures including the vagina, vaginal opening, clitoris, labia, urethra, and bladder. Rich in estrogen receptors, this system is susceptible to changes during menopause and postmenopause when estrogen levels decrease. Because estrogen is important for maintaining tissue integrity and blood flow, dropping estrogen levels can inhibit the ability of these tissues to stretch and lead to increased fragility and dryness. The resulting symptoms—collectively referred to as genitourinary syndrome of menopause (GSM)—may include vaginal dryness (the number one symptom), pain with sex, pain or burning of the vulva, a change in discharge and odor, a sandpaper-like feeling, burning with urination, increased urinary urgency, and bladder infections. GSM is incredibly common and interferes with many people's comfort and sex lives after menopause.

But, as Dr. Jen Gunter points out in *The Vagina Bible*, "There is a culture of silence about aging vulvas and vaginas. Society wants us to be doting grandmothers and eccentric detectives," so it can be challenging to get the information we need about common conditions like GSM. Even though there is great evidence for the grandmother hypothesis, that doesn't mean you must become a one-dimensional "doting grandmother" after menopause. The grandmother hypothesis just provides more evidence that we're still extremely capable and important during our postmenopausal years. We should also enjoy a sandpaper-free vagina and pain-free sex if we so choose. So what can we do if we experience GSM?

CONTINUES

Here are some treatment and care recommendations from Dr. Gunter:

- **DECREASE AGGRAVATION:** Using plain water to rinse your vulva is great, or if you want, you can use gentle cleansers like facial cleansers (just don't use ones with salicylic acid). Avoid harsh, scented soaps (which can be drying); intimate wipes that may irritate your skin; and in the case of urinary incontinence, use incontinence pads, not menstrual pads.

- **PRESERVE INTEGRITY:** Apply a natural moisturizer like coconut oil or olive oil to your vulva; consider using a pubic hair trimmer instead of waxing, as pubic hair increases humidity and keeps moisture close to the vulva.

- **CONSIDER TOPICAL ESTROGEN OR VAGINAL DHEA:** Vaginal estrogen is the gold standard for GSM. Systemic estrogen therapy may also help GSM, but is generally less effective than topical estrogen. Vaginal DHEA, which is converted to estradiol and testosterone when absorbed, is another treatment option.

After we've said goodbye to our menstrual cycles and found a home in this new version of ourselves, some people feel a sense of discovering who they truly are and their purpose in life. We may find that we are better able to create boundaries and feel less fear about what others think about us. It's as if the filter we've lived with our whole lives comes off and we're finally free to be ourselves. There's a sense of liberation after menopause, that is, as Alexandra Pope says, about "stepping up to a new level of power" and "a graduation to a new place to speak from." To step into these years with our full mental and physical power, we need to continually nurture our health. There is a word that scientists use to describe people who are exceptionally good at remaining sharp and healthy well into older age—"superagers."

Grit and Good Stress

If "feminine forever" is like a serum you buy that (falsely) promises to make you look and feel twenty years younger (along with promoting other stereotypical ideals of femininity), superaging is like a magical cape that says, "Who cares about wrinkles? I'm here to fly!" In the most basic terms, superagers are people who are good at aging. They are sixty to eighty years old, and their memories are equal to or better than people twenty to thirty years younger. According to Lisa Feldman Barrett, superagers consistently challenge themselves mentally and physically with new things outside of their comfort zone.

We might think of menopause and our postmenopausal years as an initiation to traveling outside of our comfort zone to a new bodily landscape, hormonal milieu, and season of life. During this time of flux and recalibration, we may ditch some of our old patterns that aren't serving us and find ourselves in new terrain with a refreshed sense of purpose. How we feel during this time in our lives is highly reflective of how well we've taken care of ourselves, and how we've managed our stress, the last few decades. Throughout this book, we've revisited again and again the detrimental effects of chronic stress on our hormonal, mental, and reproductive health. Over time, chronic stress has a negative impact on certain regions in our brains. However, Barrett points out that we do need some stress, specifically the kind of good stress that shows up when we're challenged, to keep our brains healthy. When we're mentally or physically challenged, we're asking our brains to work harder. In superagers, certain regions of the brain are thicker and better connected including the anterior insula, the hippocampus, the medial prefrontal cortex, and others.

These brain regions, which Barrett dubs the "superager ensemble," keep us alive, and of equal importance, healthy. To do this, our brains need us to work through discomfort and exertion and this takes "grit." The psychologist Angela Duckworth uses this word to describe the motivation required to persevere through uncomfortable challenges. In her book *Grit: The Power of Passion and Perseverance*, she describes how highly accomplished people "have no realistic expectation of ever catching up to their ambitions," and though they never believe they are good enough, importantly, they are "satisfied being unsatisfied." The kind of dogged, unrelenting determination that compels us to work toward our ambitions—even when the chase causes us pain, boredom, or frustration—fosters unusually high resilience and enduring passion. The combination of perseverance and passion, Duckworth writes, is what makes high achievers special, and it is what composes the key to that specialness: grit.

Grit puts the "super" in superagers, as these folks have a habit of pushing themselves beyond their physical and mental boundaries. Challenges that force us, in a literal sense, to grow tend to come with heaping servings of self-doubt, frustration, failure, and feelings of defeat, but getting our grit on and working through these feelings strengthen our superager ensemble. What these experiences and challenges do is preserve neuroanatomical networks involved in memory encoding and retrieval along with cognitive and executive functioning, which appear to protect us from developing dementia. As discussed in the last chapter, we lose some of the neuroprotective benefits of estrogen during and after menopause, which may induce brain changes that put us at higher risk for developing diseases like Alzheimer's. Along with eating nutrient-dense foods and practicing self-care, cultivating physical and mental grit are some of the most important and effective ways that we can modify that risk.

However, grit isn't the only essential ingredient for cognitive health. In *The Extended Mind: The Power of Thinking Outside the Brain*, the science writer Annie Murphy Paul details the way our brains use the body, the spaces around us, and other people to think. She explores these three categories, also known as embodied cognition (think movements such as walking and hand gestures), situated cognition (how our surroundings such as nature and built environments affect thinking), and distributed cognition (how we think with others in a group), to challenge our "brain bound" culture that leaves out how reliant our cognition is on the world around us. Some of the practical and applicable at any age principles she recommends include checking in with our physical sensations, or body budget, presented in the last chapter (see page 222), daily movement like walking, which is especially generative if done in green spaces and/or with company as this promotes synchronized movement—another action that benefits our thinking. She also recommends offloading information to free up cognitive space through the practice of journaling and talking out or constructively arguing out ideas with others to work through problems. These actions (and many others she writes about) generate cognitive loops wherein an idea or problem starts in the brain and then gets circulated out into the world through embodied, situated, or distributed cognition, then reenters the brain, then goes back out into the world again, and so on. Our brains love this loopiness in cognition—a kind of inhale and exhale for our thinking patterns that allow us to revisit and revise our work and ideas in a way that is both visceral and cerebral.

Extending our thinking with the kind of extra-neural resources that Paul writes about is one way to counteract the dark side of grit that we might call "stubbornness." If grit is a rational action that moves us closer to where we want to go, stubbornness is an irrational action akin to beating our heads against a brick wall. In general, it's hard to know in the moment if we're being gritty or obstinate. Usually, we figure this out retrospectively when we're able to reflect on our past actions. Other good ways to nurture our grit, instead of our stubbornness, are to combine it with a few types of learning that contribute to long-term intellectual and cognitive health.

The neuroscientist Rachel Wu and her colleagues propose six essential factors for ongoing intellectual engagement. They are:

1. A serious commitment to learning (persevering toward mastery versus dabbling or hobby learning).

2. Learning many things at the same time.

3. A "growth mindset," the belief that our abilities aren't fixed, rather they improve with time and effort.

4. A forgiving environment that allows for mistakes and encourages trying and trying again.

5. Individualized scaffolding, or increasing the difficulty of what you're learning in response to your abilities.

6. Open-minded input-driven learning (my personal favorite), which involves observing and learning from patterns in our environment more often than we rely on knowledge and assumptions formed from previous experiences. Any activity that simultaneously deceases routines while increasing our exposure to novel tasks and environments outside our comfort zone is an example of open-minded input-driven learning. Learning a foreign language in a new country is a classic example.

If these six factors made you think of how babies and children learn, you're right on track. Wu and her colleagues developed this six-factor framework based on how prevalent these learning types are when we're young and how they tend to decline as we age. The authors argue that as we age, there is a decrease in the six factors because we tend to specialize, and the goal of specialization, or perceptual narrowing, is to apply what we've already learned to unknown situations to save time and energy. On the other hand, broad learning is about learning new skills to adapt to new environments, and the six factors promote this kind of learning. Of course, throughout our lives, there is a trade-off between specialized knowledge and broad learning. But as we age, we tend to tip the scales more toward specialization, which inherently means we become less and less able to adapt to new environments and this might put what the authors call "brakes" on our cognitive development that trigger cognitive aging whereas the six factors act more like accelerators for cognitive engagement that slow age-related cognitive decline.

In her piece in *The New Yorker*, "Is It Really Too Late to Learn New Skills?" Margaret Talbot wrote that broad learning, also called "fluid intelligence," favors the young who are able to quickly adapt to their environment and think on their feet. On the other hand, "crystallized intelligence," aka specialized knowledge, favors those of older age and allows us to tap into what we already know to navigate situations. We reap the cognitive benefits when we balance both types of learning. We can look forward to increased crystallized knowledge and, Talbot writes, social understanding, while also making an effort to remain fluid and adaptable.

What to Expect When You're Expecting

Imagine preparing for the menopausal transition and postmenopausal years like we prepare for childbirth, but instead, think of it as your own rebirth. The gestation period is much longer and occurs during our late reproductive years. We know a major transition is coming, that it might not be easy, and that after, life will never be the same. So we thoroughly educate ourselves, learning from people in our culture and others, about how to navigate this transition the best that we can. We find an excellent provider and support team and nurture ourselves with food, movement, and self-care. What we know about childbirth is what we also know about menopause: menopause is not an end, but a new beginning. Research shows that people who fear childbirth tend to experience significantly higher anxiety during pregnancy, have negative birth experiences, and continue feeling negative about their birth experiences long after the birth is over. In that situation, what helps shift perception from negative to positive and decrease fear is becoming confident in reproductive knowledge, witnessing others give birth, and learning about pregnancy and birth through friends.

These three factors—confidence in our knowledge, acting as a witness, and learning from others—are so powerful because they allow us to reclaim our experiences from medicalization and mass-mediated information and act as a gateway to empowerment. These factors translate to each phase, season, and cycle of life. They connect us to the unknown, reducing our fear and replacing helplessness with a deep understanding that, throughout our lifespans and especially at the end, we are as valuable and essential as the Hadza and orca grandmothers who keep future generations alive with their deep care, ecological knowledge, and grit.

Movement and Self-Care

Practice Quality Movement

Moving is about maintaining autonomy and function, reducing pain, and feeling capable and self-reliant. We're not sold as many natural movement "workouts" as much as we're sold exercise because we can get natural movement for free on long walks and hikes, walking up and down stairs, sitting on the floor, shoveling snow, lifting heavy objects, squatting to garden, playing with young children, and other activities of daily life. Diverse, low-intensity movement scattered throughout our whole day instead of crammed into an hour of high-intensity exercise is one of the habits people in Blue Zones (places in the world with the highest number of centenarians) have in common. Moving more and choosing quality movement matter!

A decline in circulating estrogens following menopause is associated with increased inflammation. The higher our systemic inflammation, the more at risk we are for developing type 2 diabetes, cancer, and cardiovascular disease—the leading cause of death in postmenopausal women. A 2020 study from *Scientific Reports* examined pro-inflammatory molecules called cytokines in healthy postmenopausal women before and after twenty-four months of dietary and nutritional intervention. The cisgender women randomized to the physical activity intervention, which consisted of daily moderate-intensity physical activity along with one hour of monitored strenuous activity per week, showed lower levels of some pro-inflammatory cytokines compared to the control group, who received general recommendations to eat healthy (mostly plant foods) and exercise. The authors concluded that regular physical activity effectively reduces inflammatory markers over time and may even reduce the risk of chronic diseases in postmenopausal women. Another study found that a sedentary lifestyle, defined as walking fewer than six thousand steps a day, combined with high-carbohydrate intake was associated with cardiovascular risk and low-grade chronic inflammation in postmenopause. The takeaway from these studies? Set goals to improve how you move and keep moving your body. Maybe this means practicing getting up off the ground to a standing position, improving balance and climbing ability, and in the case of pain or injuries, finding ways to move creatively.

Power Nine

Moving naturally is just one of the nine specific lifestyle characteristics researchers identified among people who live in Blue Zones (such as Loma Linda, California; Nicoya, Costa Rica; Sardinia, Italy; Ikaria, Greece; and Okinawa, Japan). Many people in these zones make it into their nineties without chronic diseases. Here are the nine denominators residents who live in Blue Zones have in common according to a 2016 study:

1. **MOVE NATURALLY:** People in these zones don't typically go to the gym, lift weights, or run marathons, but they do live in environments that encourage them to move a lot all the time (see page 244).

2. **FIND PURPOSE:** According to the researchers, having a sense of purpose or a reason to wake up in the morning adds up to seven years to your lifespan.

3. **RELEASE STRESS:** Develop routines to reduce chronic stress. A few examples include gratitude practices, prayer, napping, and celebrating happy hour.

4. **80 PERCENT RULE:** the 2,500-year-old Confucian mantra—*haru hachi bu* (meaning, "Eat until you're 80% full")—is said before meals in Okinawa and reminds them to stop eating when they are 80 percent full.

5. **EAT MORE PLANTS:** Fava beans, black beans, soybeans, and lentils are the basis of many centenarian diets (along with fruits, vegetables, and whole grains), while meat consumption is more limited. Additionally, little to no processed food is consumed.

6. **VINO:** The majority of residents in Blue Zones are moderate drinkers, consuming around one to two drinks (think Sardinian wine) per day.

7. **BELONGING:** The majority of centenarians in these zones attend some kind of faith-based services.

8. **RELATIONSHIPS:** Staying close to family, committing to a life partner, and investing in their children with love and time are important to them.

9. **SOCIAL SUPPORT:** Friendships and positive social support keep them healthy in the long run.

Think Freedom

Westerners can learn from other cultures that are less likely to perceive menopause and postmenopausal years as a medical problem. A 2019 integrative review examined the relationship between social determinants of health and menopause and found that Mayan women gain increased status and respect with age and some Mayan groups rejoice when their menstrual cycles end. Chinese women consider menopause a rebirth and the time following a period of freedom when they can preserve the energy they previously lost to fertility and childbirth. Non-European women who either have a better attitude toward menopause or pay less attention to their symptoms experience fewer hot flashes and tend to accept menopause as a normal part of life.

As Susan P. Mattern writes, "We become non-reproductive so that we can do other things. The transition is important, but not because of the symptoms it may or may not cause us to suffer. It is important on a much larger scale, and to reduce it to a medical condition is to trivialize it." This altered perspective may help us navigate our postmenopausal years with better tools and a higher quality of life. That said, we live within our unique social and cultural context, so the experience of severe postmenopausal symptoms does not signal any kind of personal failure. Those experiencing symptoms or struggling with this transition should seek out high-quality care and treatment. To support changing our perspective and rewiring our brains, we might consider mindfulness-based cognitive behavioral therapy (CBT, see page 156). Some studies have found that CBT is an effective non-pharmacologic treatment for hot flashes, depression, sleep disturbances, and even sexual dysfunction.

Take the Miracle Drug

"Sleep is a miracle drug with no side effects," the psychologist and expert on grit Angela Duckworth writes. Every organ and system in our body requires sleep, and all are enhanced when we get enough sleep and impaired when we don't. Studies find that there is a relationship between self-control and sleep. Adults who are more self-controlled don't procrastinate at bedtime and end up going to sleep earlier and getting more sleep. We are able to practice better self-control when we implement specific strategies and plan ahead. In the neuroscientist Matthew Walker's book *Why We Sleep*, he provides twelve excellent tips for healthy sleep. We've covered some of the tips earlier in the book (see page 161), but here are a few more strategies from Walker that improve both self-control and sleep:

- Follow a sleep schedule. Waking up and going to sleep at the same time creates a sleep pattern, and we are creatures of habit. Walker recommends setting an alarm for bedtime to reinforce this habit.

- Avoid stimulating exercise in the two to three hours before bed and avoid caffeine in the afternoon (also avoid nicotine at all times and, if possible, medicines that disrupt sleep).

- Skip alcohol before bed and don't consume large quantities of food or fluids late at night.

- Take a hot bath before bed and give yourself enough time to unwind and relax so you're better prepared to fall asleep.

- Don't nap in the late afternoon, and if you're in bed and still awake after twenty minutes, or feeling anxious, get up and out of bed and read, stretch, look at the stars, meditate, take a bath, or do something else relaxing until you feel settled and sleepy.

Nutrition

The estrobolome is the aggregate of microbes within your gut microbiome that play a central role in regulating hormones such as estrogen. It affects the metabolism of estrogen and influences estrogen-dependent physiological reactions. An out-of-balance, or dysbiotic, gut microbiome has a negative effect on estrogen metabolism, which may contribute to the development of estrogen-related diseases such as breast cancer. Estrobolome disruption during the postmenopausal years is especially detrimental and associated with an increased risk of cardiovascular disease, obesity, and osteoporosis. Studies show that the reduced levels of circulating estrogens during the postmenopausal years contribute to significant changes in the gut and vaginal microbiome, increasing our risk of developing certain diseases such as endometrial cancer and metabolic issues that are common during the postmenopausal years. There is some evidence that hormone therapy can improve both gut and vaginal microbial health, and there is also limited evidence that supports the use of probiotics during this time. These treatments should be explored with a health care provider. For some people, improving the quality of their diet and lifestyle drastically improves gut health, negating the need for additional interventions. All of this is to say: your gut health is extremely important after menopause.

Eat Whole Foods

Inflammatory foods like sugar, soda, refined grains, processed foods, and conventionally raised dairy and livestock are detrimental to microbial health, so where possible, it's worth reducing or eliminating consumption of these substances. A 2019 study in the *American Journal of Clinical Nutrition* found that diets with high-glycemic loads (usually in the form of added sugars and refined carbohydrates) could be a potential risk factor for insomnia in postmenopausal women, whereas consumption of whole fruits, vegetables, and whole grains and higher intakes of fiber were significantly associated with lower reports of insomnia. Poor sleep quality is associated with insulin resistance in postmenopausal women, which leads to increased visceral fat along with body-wide metabolic issues.

Eat Nutrient-Dense Foods

A 2020 study in *Gut Microbiota* found that the Mediterranean diet led to decreased inflammation and microbiome changes including increased richness of certain bacteria while decreasing pro-inflammatory bacteria. Other studies show that higher adherence to this diet—meaning choosing to eat this way most of the time—results in higher bone mass and muscle mass in postmenopausal people and it's also linked to a lower risk of chronic diseases, cancer, diabetes, and heart disease. While other diets, like the ketogenic diet where you consume a high-fat diet and restrict carbohydrates, are starting to gain popularity and are often recommended during the menopausal transition and postmenopause, eating this way needs much more research and may increase the risk of heart disease, cancer, and osteoporosis. The benefit of leaning into a Mediterranean diet is that it's not overly restrictive and includes diverse foods that benefit gut and overall health. Here are some of the key components of eating this way:

- **HEALTHY FATS:** olives and extra virgin olive oil are consumed in abundance while saturated fats are limited.

- **HIGH-QUALITY PROTEINS:** a diverse assortment of fish and shellfish, organ meats, and wild game, beans, chickpeas, nuts, seeds, and eggs are cornerstones, while meat like beef, lamb, chicken, duck, goat, and pork are eaten in smaller portions.

- **VITAMIN AND MINERAL-RICH FOODS:** mushrooms, leafy greens, diverse and abundant fresh fruits and vegetables, spices and herbs, nuts and seeds, whole and unrefined grains.

- **PLENTIFUL VEGETABLES AND FRUITS:** cooked vegetables drizzled with olive oil along with a rainbow of raw fruits and vegetables are the key to this plant-based way of eating.

- **GRAINS:** whole grains like farro, oats, millet, buckwheat, barley, rice, wheat, polenta, and rye are staples and included in most meals.

Power Nine Lifestyle Tips

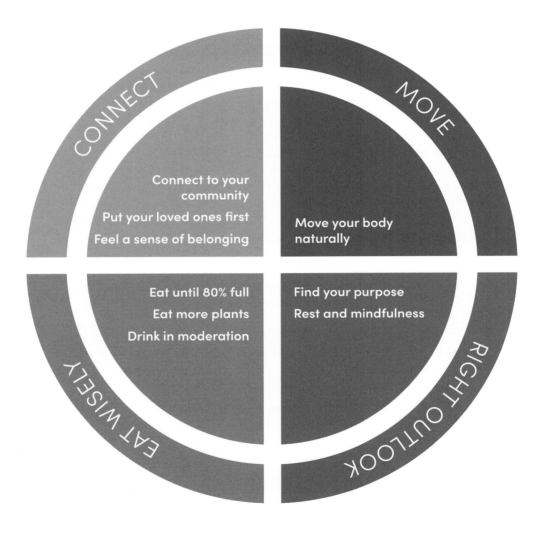

CONNECT

MOVE

Connect to your community

Put your loved ones first

Feel a sense of belonging

Move your body naturally

Eat until 80% full

Eat more plants

Drink in moderation

Find your purpose

Rest and mindfulness

EAT WISELY

RIGHT OUTLOOK

- **FERMENTED FOODS:** sauerkraut, kimchi, miso, lacto-fermented vegetables, yogurt, kefir, cheese, and other fermented dairy products feed healthy gut microbes.

- **MODERATION (EXCEPT FOR WATER!):** red wine is consumed regularly, but in small amounts (one five-ounce glass of wine daily).

- **PLEASURE:** enjoying and savoring food alone or with company—it's not just about the food, it's the whole lifestyle, see the chart.

It's Not Just Diet, It's *Diet*

As previously mentioned, the true ancient Greek definition of the word *diet* is about lifestyle as a whole including everyday choices, stress, relationships, time spent outside, and exposure to toxins. In other words, health, including and especially our microbiome health, is shaped by the interacting ecosystem that is our lifestyle. Just like people in the Blue Zones don't go to the gym to work out, they also don't subscribe to specific diet ideologies or regimens; rather, they eat close to the land and work hard to obtain, grow, and produce their own food (which I imagine they also mindfully and pleasurably consume with pleasant company). This comprehensive approach simultaneously meets all of our needs for movement, good food, and connection to both people and our environment. It's the ecological approach to a full, healthy life, and it has just a few million years of evolution behind it.

Acknowledgments

In retrospect, I can't imagine writing a book during a more challenging time. When I first started writing, I was a few weeks pregnant with my second child, editing my first book, and spending most of my time split between working in a pediatric clinic to complete my rotation for my nurse practitioner master's degree and caring for my toddler. Then, the world shut down because of the COVID-19 pandemic, and halfway through writing the book, I gave birth to my son and reentered the sleepy world of newborns and endless diapers.

What ended up happening was that everything in this book—the food, movement, and self-care—and all the scientists, writers, and advocates for people who menstruate became utterly essential for my survival and success. But even more essential to my survival and ability to string a few sentences together was my husband, Max. When I was overwhelmed, he was steady and calm. When I needed a break to get outside and into the mountains, he reached out and took our sons into his arms. And when I needed a break from the pressure and stress I was putting on myself, he was always there with a weird sexy dance, embarrassing dad joke, or charming-but-out-of-tune song. Max has the delightful ability to distract me from my work when I really need it, while also giving me abundant time and space to work. He willfully learned more about the menstrual cycle, menopausal transition, and postmenopause than he ever thought he would. There is no better person, or better partner, in the world, and I am so very grateful. Thank you, my love.

When I was writing about the grandmother hypothesis, my mom was likely holding my newborn while pushing my toddler on the swing after dropping off eggs and vegetables from her garden. Thank you, Mom, for raising me and for loving my boys. You are the most hardworking, capable, open-minded, and playful person I've ever met, and the world feels more possible and survivable with you in it. Thank you to my brother Bob. We are so fortunate that you live with us and help us raise the babies. Thanks to my brother Nick for checking in on me and encouraging my work and to my sister-in-law Mari for our conversations about womanhood and parenting. And thanks to my dad for passing down some grit (and perhaps occasional stubbornness).

I am deeply grateful for the writers, scientists, and practitioners who are champions for all women and those with ovaries and periods including Joycelyn Elders, MD; Lisa Hendrickson-Jack; Lara Briden, ND; Nicole Jardim; Erica Chidi Cohen; Angela Saini; Randi Hutter Epstein, MD; Susan P. Mattern, PhD; Florence Williams; Caroline Criado Perez; Emily Nagoski, PhD; Katy Bowman; Alexandra Pope; Sarah E. Hill, PhD; Elizabeth Kissling, PhD; Lisa Feldman Barrett, PhD; Jen Gunter, MD; Amy Tuteur, MD; Lisa Mosconi, PhD; Angela Duckworth, PhD; Kristen Hawkes, PhD; and so many more who create and share information that is trustworthy, practical, and above all, dedicated to empowering us all to make choices that improve our health and wellness while protecting our reproductive rights.

Thank you to my dear friends who talked to me about their cycles, read many drafts of this book, and offered their insight and feedback. This book is better because of all of you.

I can't imagine writing this book without the support of the whole team at Roost Books. Thank you to my editors Audra Figgins for diving into this book, reading it with incredible attention to detail, and making it so much better; and Juree Sondker, who one day many moons ago said, "What about a book about menstrual cycles?" Thank you to the team of editorial freelancers, designers, and marketers at Shambhala who are truly thoughtful, talented, and passionate creators of beautiful, meaningful books. Thank you to Cassius Adair, who helped me ensure that this book was inclusive and accessible to all people. And thank you to Dr. Johanna Koch for reviewing the science and medical information. Your honest feedback helped me write a more balanced and evidence-based book.

To my children, Holden and Otto, while you won't ever menstruate, I look forward to teaching you all about the menstrual cycle so that you may become supportive, informed, and empathetic allies for those who do.

Resources and Recommended Reading

PRODUCTS

Food

SPICES: Curio Spice Co. www.curiospice.com, Diaspora Co. www.diasporaco.com, Burlap & Barrel www.burlapandbarrel.com

HERBS: Mountain Rose Herbs www.mountainroseherbs.com, Frontier Co-op www.frontiercoop.com, Pacific Botanicals www.pacificbotanicals.com, Oshala Farm www.oshalafarm.com

BASICS (AND ELEVATED BASICS): Thrive Market www.thrivemarket.com, Well Spent Market www.wellspentmarket.com, Imperfect Foods www.imperfectfoods.com, ButcherBox www.butcherbox.com, Public Goods www.publicgoods.com, local farms and farmers' markets

Microbiome-Friendly Skin Care

Marie Veronique www.marieveronique.com, Venn Skincare www.vennskincare.com, Beekman 1802 www.beekman1802.com, Dr. Elsa Jungman www.dr-ej.com, Mother Dirt www.motherdirt.com

Movement Equipment

ZERO DROP AND MINIMALIST FOOTWEAR: Lems Shoes www.lemsshoes.com, Vivobarefoot www.vivobarefoot.com, Softstar Shoes www.softstarshoes.com, Luna Sandals www.lunasandals.com, Earth Runners www.earthrunners.com. Find them secondhand on sites like Poshmark www.poshmark.com.

NUTRITIOUS MOVEMENT EQUIPMENT SET: www.nutritiousmovement.com; half dome foam roller, yoga block, and meditation cushion: MovNat www.movnat.com.

Cycle Tracking, Menstrual, and Sexual Wellness Products (changing rapidly!)

APPS: Clue, MyFLO, Eve by Glow, Ovia, Natural Cycles, Cycle, Kindara, Flo

WEARABLE TECHNOLOGY: Ava Bracelet, Tempdrop, Wink, Yono, Daysy

SUSTAINABLE MENSTRUAL PRODUCTS: Saalt Wear Leakproof Underwear, Period Aisle Reusable Pads and Gender-Neutral Boxer Brief, Lunette Menstrual Cup, Rael Menstrual Cup and Pads, Thinx Leakproof Underwear, DivaCup, Intimina Ziggy Cup, Knix Leakproof Underwear

SEXUAL WELLNESS PRODUCTS: Sustain Natural Condoms, Glyde Condoms, Lola Condoms, Unique Plus Condoms, Lovability Condoms, Sir Richard's Condoms

BOOKS: *Fertility Awareness Mastery Charting Workbook* by Lisa Hendrickson-Jack, *Taking Charge of your Fertility: The Definitive Guide to Natural Birth Control, Pregnancy Achievement, and Reproductive Health* by Toni Weschler

Meditation and Self-Care Apps

Ten Percent Happier, Headspace, Insight Timer, Calm, Moodfit, MoodMissions, Happify, Shine

BOOKS

Movement and Nature

Grow Wild: The Whole-Child, Whole-Family, Nature-Rich Guide to Moving More by Katy Bowman

Movement Matters: Essays on Movement Science, Movement Ecology, and the Nature of Movement by Katy Bowman

The Extended Mind: The Power of Thinking Outside the Brain by Annie Murphy Paul

The Nature Fix: Why Nature Makes Us Happier, Healthier, and More Creative by Florence Williams

Self-Care, Sexuality, Menstrual Cycle, and Menopause

Aroused: The History of Hormones and How They Control Just About Everything by Randi Hutter Epstein, MD

Breasts: A Natural and Unnatural History by Florence Williams

Burnout: The Secret to Unlocking the Stress Cycle by Emily Nagoski and Amelia Nagoski

Come as You Are: The Surprising New Science That Will Transform Your Sex Life by Emily Nagoski, PhD

Fix Your Period: Six Weeks to Banish Bloating, Conquer Cramps, Manage Moodiness, and Ignite Lasting Hormone Balance by Nicole Jardim

Hormone Repair Manual: Every Woman's Guide to Healthy Hormones After 40 by Lara Briden, ND

Menopocalypse: How I Learned to Thrive During Menopause and How You Can Too by Amanda Thebe

Period Power: A Manifesto for the Menstrual Movement by Nadya Okamoto

Period Power: Harness Your Hormones and Get Your Cycle Working for You by Maisie Hill

Period Repair Manual: Natural Treatment for Better Hormones and Better Periods by Lara Briden, ND

The Birth of the Pill: How Four Crusaders Reinvented Sex and Launched a Revolution by Jonathan Eig

The Extended Mind: The Power of Thinking Outside the Brain by Annie Murphy Paul

The Fifth Vital Sign: Master your Cycles & Optimize Your Fertility by Lisa Hendrickson-Jack

The Menopause Manifesto: Own Your Health with Facts and Feminism by Jen Gunter, MD

The Palgrave Handbook of Critical Menstruation Studies edited by Chris Bobel, Inga T. Winkler, Breanne Fahs, Katie Hasson, Elizabeth Arveda Kissling, and Tomi Ann Roberts

The Slow Moon Climbs: The Science, History, and Meaning of Menopause by Susan P. Mattern, PhD

The Vagina Bible: The Vulva and The Vagina—Separating the Myth from the Medicine by Jen Gunter, MD

References

CHAPTER 1
YOUR CYCLE MATTERS

Alvergne, Alexandra, and Vedrana Högqvist Tabor. "Is Female Health Cyclical? Evolutionary Perspectives on Menstruation." *Trends in Ecology & Evolution* 33, no. 6 (2018): 399–414. doi.org/10.1016/j.tree.2018.03.006.

Druet, Anna. "How Did Menstruation Become Taboo?" Hello Clue, May 4, 2021. helloclue.com/articles/culture/how-did-menstruation-become-taboo.

Emera, Deena, Roberto Romero, and Günter Wagner. "The Evolution of Menstruation: A New Model for Genetic Assimilation: Explaining Molecular Origins of Maternal Responses to Fetal Invasiveness." *BioEssays* 34, no. 1 (2012): 26–35. doi.org/10.1002/bies.201100099.

Knight, Chris. *Blood Relations: Menstruation and the Origins of Culture*. Connecticut: Yale University Press, 1995.

Okada, Hidetaka, Tomoko Tsuzuki, and Hiromi Murata. "Decidualization of the Human Endometrium." *Reproductive Medicine and Biology* 17, no.3 (2018): 220–27. doi.org/10.1002/rmb2.12088.

Shtulman, Andrew, and Laura Schulz. "The Relation Between Essentialist Beliefs and Evolutionary Reasoning." *Cognitive Science* 32, no. 6 (2008): 1049–62. doi.org/10.1080/03640210801897864.

Vigil, Pilar, Carolina Lyon, Betsi Flores, Hernan Rioseco, and Felipe Serrano. "Ovulation, A Sign of Health." *Linacre Quarterly* 84, no. 4 (2017): 343–55. doi.org/10.1080/00243639.2017.1394053.

Winkler, Inga T. "Introduction: Menstruation as Fundamental." In *The Palgrave Handbook of Critical Menstruation Studies*, edited by Chris Bobel, Inga T. Winkler, Breanne Fahs, Katie Ann Hasson, Elizabeth Arveda Kissling, and Tomi-Ann Roberts, 9–13. Singapore: Palgrave Macmillan, 2020.

CHAPTER 2
THE NAMING OF *ELIXIR VITAE*

Acevedo-Rodriquez, A., A. S. Kauffman, B. D. Cherrington, C. S. Borges, T. A. Roepke, and M. Laconi. "Emerging Insights into Hypothalamic-Pituitary-Gonadal Axis Regulation and Interaction with Stress Signaling." *Journal of Neuroendocrinology* 30, no. 10 (2018): e12590. doi.org/10.1111/jne.12590.

Berg, Erika Gebel. "The Chemistry of the Pill," *ACS Central Science* 1, no. 1 (2015): 5–7. doi.org/10.1021/acscentsci.5b00066.

Chidi-Ogbolu, Nkechinyere, and Keith Baar. "Effect of Estrogen on Musculoskeletal Performance and Injury Risk." *Frontiers in Physiology* 9, no. 1834 (2019). doi.org/10.3389/phys.2018.01834.

Eig, Jonathan. *The Birth of the Pill: How Four Crusaders Reinvented Sex and Launched a Revolution.* New York: W. W. Norton, 2015.

Epstein, Randi Hutter. *Aroused: The History of Hormones and How They Control Just About Everything.* New York: W. W. Norton, 2018.

González-Orozco, Juan Carlos, and Ignacio Camacho-Arroyo. "Progesterone Actions During Central Nervous System Development." *Frontiers of Neuroscience* 13, no. 503 (2019). doi.org/10.3389/fnins.2019.00503.

Hill, Sarah E. *This is Your Brain on Birth Control: The Surprising Science of Women, Hormones, and the Law of Unintended Consequences.* New York: Avery, 2019.

Joseph, Dana N., and Shannon Whirledge. "Stress and the HPA Axis: Balancing Homeostasis and Fertility." *International Journal of Molecular Science* 18, no. 10 (2017): 2224. doi.org/10.3390/ijms18102224.

La Merrill, Michele A., Laura N. Vandenberg, Martyn T. Smith, William Goodson, Patience Browne, Heather B. Patisaul, Kathryn Z. Guyton et al. "Consensus on the Key Characteristics of Endocrine-Disrupting Chemicals as a Basis for Hazard Identification." *Nature Reviews Endocrinology* 16, no. 1 (2020): 45–57. doi.org/10.1038/s41574-019-0273-8.

Lauretta, Rosa, Andrea Sansone, Massimiliano Sansone, Francesco Romanelli, and Marialuisa Appetecchia. "Endocrine Disrupting Chemicals: Effects of Endocrine Glands." *Frontiers in Endocrinology* 10, no. 178 (2019). doi.org/10.3389/fendo.2019.00178.

Liao, Pamela Verma, and Janet Dollin. "Half a Century of the Oral Contraceptive Pill: Historical Review and View to the Future." *Canadian Family Physician* 58, no. 12 (2012): e757–60. ncbi.nlm.nih.gov/pmc/articles/PMC3520685/pdf/058e757.pdf.

Morgenroth, Thekla, and Michelle K. Ryan. "The Effects of Gender Trouble: An Integrative Theoretical Framework of the Perpetuation and Disruption of the Gender/Sex Binary," *Perspectives on Psychological Science* 16, no. 6(2020): 1113–42. doi.org/10.1177/1745691620902442.

Nagoski, Emily. *Come As You Are: The Surprising New Science That Will Transform Your Sex Life*. New York: Simon & Schuster, 2015.

Nussey, Stephen, and Saffron Whitehead. *Endocrinology: An Integrated Approach*. Oxford: BIOS Scientific Publishers, 2001.

Oyola, Mario G., and Robert J. Handa. "Hypothalamic-Pituitary-Adrenal and Hypothalamic-Pituitary-Gonadal Axes: Sex Differences in Regulation of Stress Responsivity." *Stress* 20, no. 5 (2017): 476–94. doi.org/10.1080/10253890.2017.1369523.

Reed, Beverly G., Bruce R. Carr et al. "The Normal Menstrual Cycle and the Control of Ovulation." In *Endotext*. Massachusetts: MDText.com, Inc. 2018. ncbi.nlm.nih.gov/books/NBK279054.

Rettberg, Jamaica R., Jia Yao, and Roberta Diaz Brinton. "Estrogen: A Master Regulator of Bioenergetic Systems in the Brain and Body," *Frontiers in Neuroendocrinology* 35, no. 1 (2014): 8–30. doi.org/10.1016/j.yfrne.2013.08.001.

Ruiz, Daniel, Marisol Becerra, Jyotsna S. Jagai, Kerry Ard, and Robert M. Sargis. "Disparities in Environmental Exposures to Endocrine-Disrupting Chemicals and Diabetes Risk in Vulnerable Populations," *Diabetes Care* 41, no. 1 (2018): 193–205. doi.org/10.2337/dc16-2765.

Saini, Angela. *Inferior: How Science Got Women Wrong and the New Research That's Rewriting the Story*. Boston: Beacon Press, 2016.

Taraborrelli, Stefania. "Physiology, Production and Action of Progesterone." *Acta Obstetricia et Gynecologica Scandinavica* 94, no. S161 (2015): 8–16. doi.org/10.1111.aogs.12771.

Tata, Jamshed R. "One Hundred Years of Hormones," *EMBO Reports* 6 (2005): 490–96. doi.org/10.1038/sj.embor.7400444.

Tippett, Krista. "Alain de Botton: The True Hard Work of Love and Relationships." *On Being*. February 11, 2021. onbeing.org/programs/alain-de-botton-the-true-hard-work-of-love-and-relationships.

Wessels, Jocelyn M., Allison M. Felker, Haley A. Dupont, and Charu Kaushic. "The Relationship Between Sex Hormones, The Vaginal Microbiome and Immunity in HIV-1 Susceptibility in Women." *Disease Models and Mechanisms* 11, no. 9 (2018). doi. org/10.1242/dmm.035147.

Young, Lauren J. "Your Cervical Mucus is Beautiful." *Science Friday*. February 4, 2020. sciencefriday.com/articles/cervical-mucus-health.

CHAPTER 3
THE CYCLE AND THE BRAIN

Bittel, Carla. *Mary Putnam Jacobi: And the Politics of Medicine in Nineteenth-Century America*. Chapel Hill: University of North Carolina Press, 2020.

Derntl, Birgit, Ramona L. Hack, Ilse Krypsin-Exner, and Ute Habel. "Association of Menstrual Cycle Phase with the Core Components of Empathy." *Hormones and Behavior* 63, no. 1 (2013): 97–104. doi.org/10.1016/j.yhbeh.2012.10.009.

Fleischman, Diana S., and Daniel M. T. Fessler. "Progesterone's Effects on the Psychology of Disease Avoidance: Support for the Compensatory Behavioral Prophylaxis Hypothesis." *Hormones and Behavior* 59, no. 2 (2011): 271–75. doi. org/10.1016/j.yhbeh.2010.11.014.

Hyde, Janet Shibley. "The Gender Similarities Hypothesis." *American Psychologist* 60, no. 6 (2005): 581–92. doi.org/10.1037/0003-066X.60.6.581.

Le, Jessica, Natalie Thomas, and Caroline Gurvich. "Cognition, The Menstrual Cycle, and Premenstrual Disorders: A Review." *Brain Sciences* 10, no. 4 (2020): 198. doi. org/10.3390/brainsci10040198.

Leeners, Brigitte, Tillmann H. C. Kruger, Kirsten Geraedts, Enrico Tronci, Toni Mancini, Fabian Ille, Marcel Egli et al. "Lack of Associations Between Female Hormone Levels and Visuospatial Working Memory, Divided Attention and Cognitive Bias Across Two Consecutive Menstrual Cycles." *Frontiers in Behavioral Neuroscience* 11, no. 120 (2017). doi.org/10.3389/fnbeh.2017.00120.

Lorenz, Tierney K., Gregory E. Demas, and Julia R. Heiman. "Partnered Sexual Activity Moderates Menstrual Cycle-Related Changes in Inflammation Markers in Healthy Women: An Exploratory Observational Study." *Fertility and Sterility* 107, no. 3 (2017): 763–73. doi.org/10.1016/j.fertnstert.2016.11.010.

Lorenz, Tierney K., Carol M. Worthman, and Virginia J. Vitzhum. "Links Among Inflammation, Sexual Activity and Ovulation: Evolutionary Trade-Offs and Clinical Implications." *Evolution, Medicine, and Public Health* 2015, no.1, (2015): 304–24. doi. org/10.1093/emph/eov029.

Nielsen, Shawn E., Imran Ahmed, and Larry Cahill. "Sex and Menstrual Cycle Phase at Encoding Influence Emotional Memory for Gist and Detail." *Neurobiology of Learning and Memory* 106 (2013): 56–65. doi.org/10.1016/j.nlm.2013.07.015.

Rybaczyk, Leszek A., Meredith J. Bashaw, Dorothy R. Pathak, Scott M. Moody, Roger M. Gilders, and Donald L. Holzschu. "An Overlooked Connection: Serotonergic Mediation of Estrogen-Related Physiology and Pathology." *BMC Women's Health* 5, no. 12 (2005). doi.org/10.1186/1472-6874/5/12.

Sundström, Inger P., and Malin Gingnell. "Menstrual Cycle Influence on Cognitive Functioning and Emotion Processing—From a Reproductive Perspective." *Frontiers in Neuroscience* 8, no. 380 (2014). doi.org/10.3389/fnins.2014.00380.

CHAPTER 4
EAT, MOVE, (SELF) LOVE

Ahmed, E. M., and Marwa Al-Moghazy. "Microbial Endocrinology: Interaction of the Microbial Hormones with the Host." *Biomedical Journal of Scientific & Technical Research* 24, no. 2 (2020). doi.org/10.26717/BJSTR.2020.24.004015.

Alcock, Joe, Carlo C. Maley, and C. Athena Aktipis. "Is Eating Behavior Manipulated by the Gastrointestinal Microbiota? Evolutionary Pressures and Potential Mechanisms." *BioEssays* 36, no. 10 (2014): 940–49. doi.org/10.1002/bies.201400071.

Brown, Tracey J., Julii Brainard, Fujian Song, Xia Wang, Asmaa Abdelhamid, and Lee Hooper. "Omega 3, Omega-6, and Total Dietary Polyunsaturated Fat for Prevention and Treatment of Type 2 Diabetes Mellitus: Systematic Review and Meta-Analysis of Randomized Controlled Trials." *BMJ* 366, no. l4697 (2019). doi.org/10.1136/bmj.l4697.

Bryant, Richard A., Kim L. Felmingham, Derrick Silove, Mark Creamer, Meaghan O'Donnell, Alexander C. McFarlane. "The Associations Between Menstrual Cycle and Traumatic Memories." *Journal of Affective Disorders* 131, no. 1–3 (2011): 398–401. doi. org/10.1016/j.jad.2010.10.049.

Cai, Xiaoyan, Yunlong Zhang, Meijun Li, Jason Hy Wu, Linlin Mai, Jun Li, and Yu Yang et al. "Association Between Prediabetes and Risk of All Cause Mortality and Cardiovascular Disease: Updated Meta-Analysis." *BMJ* 370, no. m2297 (2020). doi. org/10.1136/bmj.m2297.

Chang, Courtney R., Monique E. Francois, and Jonathan P. Little. "Restricting Carbohydrates at Breakfast is Sufficient to Reduce 24-hour Postprandial Hyperglycemia and Improve Glycemic Variability." *The American Journal of Clinical Nutrition* 109, no. 5 (2019): 1302–09. doi.org/10.1093/ajcn/nqy261.

Dominianni, Christine, Rashmi Sinha, James J. Goedert, Zhiheng Pei, Liying Yang, Richard B. Hayes, and Jiyoung Ahn. "Sex, Body Mass Index, and Dietary Fiber Intake Influence the Human Gut Microbiome." *PLOS One* 10, no. 4 (2015). doi.org/10.1371/journal.pone.0124599.

Forouhi, Nita G., Anoop Misra, Viswanathan Mohan, Roy Taylor, and William Yancy. "Dietary and Nutritional Approaches for Prevention and Management of Type 2 Diabetes." *BMJ* 361, no. k2234 (2019). doi.org/10.1136/bmj.k2234.

Galicia-Garcia, Unai, Asier Benito-Vicente, Shifa Jebari, Asier Larrea-Sebal, Haziq Siddiqi, Kepa B. Uribe, Helena Ostolaza, and César Martín. "Pathophysiology of Type 2 Diabetes Mellitus." *International Journal of Molecular Sciences* 21, no. 17 (2020): 6275. doi.org/10.3390/ijms21176275.

Gelder, Sarah van. "The Radical Work of Healing: Fania and Davis on a New Kind of Civil Rights Activism." *Yes! Solutions Journalism.* February 19, 2016. yesmagazine.org/issue/life-after-oil/2016/02/19/the-radical-work-of-healing-fania-and-angela-davis-on-a-new-kind-of-civil-rights-activism.

Holick, Michael F. "Vitamin D Status: Measurement, Interpretation, and Clinical Application." *Annals of Epidemiology* 19, no. 2 (2009): 73–78. doi.org/10.1016/j.anneepidem.2007.12.001.

Hölzel, Britta K., James Carmody, Mark Vangel, Christina Congleton, Sita M. Yerramsetti, Tim Gard, and Sara W. Lazar. "Mindfulness Practice Leads to Increases in Regional Brain Gray Matter Density." *Psychiatry Research* 191, no. 1 (2011): 36–43. doi.org/10.1016/j.pscychresns.2010.08.006.

Hyde, Janet Shibley. "The Gender Similarities Hypothesis." *American Psychologist* 60, no. 6 (2005): 581–92. doi.org/10.1037/0003-066X.60.6.581.

Knoll, Jessica. "Smash the Wellness Industry." *New York Times*, June 8, 2019. nytimes.com/2019/06/08/opinion/sunday/women-dieting-wellness.html.

Łagowska, Karolina. "The Relationship Between Vitamin D Status and the Menstrual Cycle in Young Women: A Preliminary Study." *Nutrients* 10, no. 11 (2018): 1729. doi.org/10.3390/nu10111729.

Le, Jessica, Natalie Thomas, and Caroline Gurvich. "Cognition, The Menstrual Cycle, and Premenstrual Disorders: A Review." *Brain Sciences* 10, no. 4 (2020): 198. doi.org/10.3390/brainsci10040198.

Mauvais-Jarvis, Franck, Deborah Clegg, and Andrea L. Hevener. "The Role of Estrogens in Control of Energy Balance and Glucose Homeostasis. *Endocrine Reviews* 34, no. 3 (2013): 309–38. doi.org/10.1210/er.2012-1055.

Rachdaoui, Nadia, and Dipak K. Sarkar. "Effects of Alcohol on the Endocrine System." *Endocrinology Metabolism Clinic North America* 42, no. 3 (2013): 593–615. doi.org/10.1016/j.ecl.2013.05.008.

Rowe, Melissah, Liisa Veerus, Pål Trosvik, Angus Buckling, and Tommaso Pizzari. "The Reproductive Microbiome: An Emerging Driver of Sexual Selection, Sexual Conflict, Mating Systems, and Reproductive Isolation." *Trends in Ecology & Evolution* 35, no. 3 (2020): 220–34. doi.org/10.1016/j.tree.2019.11.004.

Ryan, Timothy M., and Colin N. Shaw. "Gracility of the Modern *Homo Sapiens* Skeleton is the Result of Decreased Biomechanical Loading." *Proceedings of the National Academy of Sciences* 112, no. 2 (2014): 372–77. doi.org/10.1073/pnas.1418646112.

Saif-Elnasr, Mostafa, Iman M. Ibrahim, and Manal M. Alkady. "Role of Vitamin D on Glycemic Control and Oxidative Stress in Type 2 Diabetes Mellitus." *Journal of Research in Medical Sciences* 22 (2017): 22. doi.org/10.4103/1735-1995.200278.

Samadi, Zeinab, Farzaneh Taghian, and Mahboubeh Valiani. "The Effects of Eight Weeks of Regular Aerobic Exercise on the Symptoms of Premenstrual Syndrome in Non-Athlete Girls." *Iranian Journal of Nursing and Midwifery Research* 18, no. 1 (2013): 14–19. ncbi.nlm.nih.gov/pmc/articles/PMC3748549/.

Trico, D., E. Filice, S. Trifiro, and A. Natali. "Manipulating the Sequence of Food Ingestion Improves Glycemic Control in Type 2 Diabetic Patients Under Free-Living Conditions." *Nutrition & Diabetes* 6, no. 8 (2016): e226. doi.org/10.1038/nutd.2016.33.

Tsiompanou, Eleni, and Spyros G. Marketos. "Hippocrates: Timeless Still." *Journal of the Royal Society of Medicine* 106, no. 7 (2013): 288–92. doi.org/10.1177/0141076813492945.

Vieira-Potter, Victoria J. "Effects of Sex Hormones and Exercise on Adipose Tissue." Edited by Anthony C. Hackney. *Sex Hormones, Exercise and Women.* (2017): 257–84. doi.org/10.1007/978-3-319-44558-8_15.

CHAPTER 5
A BRIEF HISTORY OF CONTRACEPTION AND THE MODERN OPTIONS

Baker, Fiona C., and Helen S. Driver. "Cicardian Rhythms, Sleep, and the Menstrual Cycle." *Sleep Medicine* 8, no. 6 (2007): 613–22. doi.org/10.1016/j.sleep.2006.09.011.

Charkoudian, Nisha, and Nina S. Stachenfeld. "Reproductive Hormone Influences on Thermoregulation in Women." *Comprehensive Physiology* 4, no. 2 (2014): 793–804. doi.org/10.1002/cphy.c130029.

Druet, Anna. "How Does Discharge Change Across the Cycle?" Hello Clue, July 10, 2019. helloclue.com/articles/cycle-a-z/wet-sticky-what-your-discharge-is-telling-you.

Hendrickson-Jack, Lisa. *The Fifth Vital Sign: Master Your Cycles & Optimize Your Fertility.* USA: Fertility Friday Publishing Inc., 2019.

Khan, Fahd, Saheel Mukhtar, Ian K. Dickinson, and Seshadri Sriprasad. "The Story of the Condom." *Indian Journal of Urology* 29, no. 1 (2013): 12–15. doi.org/10.4103/0970-1591.109976.

Knight, Jane. *The Complete Guide to Fertility Awareness.* New York: Routledge, 2017.

Lieberman, Hallie. "A Short History of the Condom." *JSTOR Daily*, June 8, 2017. daily.jstor.org/short-history-of-the-condom.

Otai, Jane. "No, Drinking Hot Water or Jumping Vigorously After Sex Won't Prevent Pregnancy." *HUB John Hopkins University*, February 1, 2016. hub.jhu.edu/2016/02/01/teen-pregnancy-contraception-in-africa.

Prather, Cynthia, Taleria R. Fuller, Khiya J. Marshall, and William L. Jeffries. "The Impact of Racism on the Sexual and Reproductive Health of African American Women." *Journal of Women's Health (Larchmt)* 25, no. 7 (2016): 664–71. doi.org/10.1089/jwh.2015.5637.

Pyper, Cecilia M. M., and Jane Knight. "Fertility Awareness Methods of Family Planning for Achieving or Avoiding Pregnancy." *The Global Library of Women's Medicine* (2008). doi.org/10.3843/GLOWM.10384.

CHAPTER 6
MENSTRUAL PHASE

Borunda, Alejandra. "How Tampons and Pads Became So Unsustainable." *National Geographic*, September 6, 2019. nationalgeographic.com/environment/2019/09/how-tampons-pads-became-unsustainable-story-of-plastic.

Boutot, Maegan. "Cycle Science: Hormonal Contraception and Your Body." *Medium*, January 6, 2017). medium.com/clued-in/cycle-science-hormonal-contraception-and-your-body-52d204137921.

Bull, Jonathan R., Simon P. Rowland, Elina B. Scherwitzl, Raoul Scherwitzl, Kristina G. Danielsson, and Joyce Harper. "Real-World Menstrual Cycle Characteristics of More Than 600,000 Menstrual Cycles." *npj Digital Medicine* 2, no. 83 (2019). doi.org/10.1038/s41746-019-0152-7.

Chen, Lijun, Jingjing Qu, and Charlie Xiang. "The Multi-Functional Roles of Menstrual Blood-Derived Stem Cells in Regenerative Medicine." *Stem Cells Research & Therapy* 10, no. 1 (2019). doi.org/10.1186/s13287-018-1105-9.

Chen, X. Chen, Claire B. Draucker, and Janet S. Carpenter. "What Women Say About Their Dysmenorrhea: A Qualitative Thematic Analysis." *BMC Women's Health* 18, no. 1 (2018): 47. doi.org/10.1186/s12905-018-0538-8.

Dmitrović, Romana. "Transvaginal Color Doppler Study of Uterine Blood Flow in Primary Dysmenorrhea." *Acta Obstetricia et Gynecologica Scandinavica* 79, no. 12 (2000): 1112–16. doi.org/10.1034/j.1600-0412.2000.0790121112.x.

Jo, Junyoung, and Sun Haeng Lee. "Heat Therapy for Primary Dysmenorrhea: A Systematic Review and Meta-Analysis of its Effects on Pain Relief and Quality of Life." *Scientific Reports* 8, no. 1 (2018): 16252. doi.org/1038/s41598-018-34303-z.

Kissling, Elizabeth A. "Bleeding Out Loud: Communication About Menstruation." *Feminism & Psychology* 6, no. 4. (1996): 481–504. doi.org/10.1177/0959353596064002.

Kissling, Elizabeth A. "Is PMS Overblown?" *Ms. Magazine*, October 23, 2012. msmagazine.com/2012/10/23/is-pms-overblown-thats-what-research-shows.

Maybin, Jacqueline A., and Hilary O. D. Critchley. "Menstrual Physiology: Implications for Endometrial Pathology and Beyond." *Human Reproduction Update* 21, no. 6 (2015): 748–61. doi.org/10.1093/humupd/dmv038.

Nadeau, Marie-Véronique. *Acne Answer*. Altadena, CA: Bitingduck Press, 2016.

Najafi, Nastaran, Hamidreza Khalkhali, Fatemeh M. Tabrizi, and Rasoul Zarrin. "Major Dietary Patterns in Relation to Menstrual Pain: A Nested Case Control Study." *BMC Women's Health* 18, no. 1 (2018): 69. doi.org/10.1186/s12905-018-0558-4.

Odell, Jenny. *How to Do Nothing: Resisting the Attention Economy*. New York: Melville House, 2019.

Palomba, Stefano, Jessica Daolio, Sara Romeo, Francesco Antonino Battaglia, Roberto Marci, and Giovanni Battista La Sala. "Lifestyle and Fertility: The Influence of Stress and Quality of Life on Female Fertility." *Reproductive Biology and Endocrinology* 16 (2018): 113. doi.org/10.1186/s12958-018-0434-y.

Park, Chan Jin, Radwa Barakat, Alexander Ulanov, Zhong Li, Po-Ching Lin, Karen Chiu, Sherry Zhou et al. "Sanitary Pads and Diapers Contain Higher Phthalate Contents Than Those in Common Commercial Plastic Products." *Reproductive Toxicology* 84 (2019): 114–21. doi.org/10.1016/j.reprotox.2019.01.005.

Raghunath, R. S., Z. C. Venables, and G. W. M. Millington. "The Menstrual Cycle and the Skin." *Clinical Dermatology* 40, no. 2 (2015): 111–15. doi.org/10.1111/ced.12588.

Saleh, Hend S., Hala E. Mowafy, and Azza A. abd El Hameid. "Stretching or Core Strengthening Exercises for Managing Primary Dysmenorrhea." *Journal of Women's Health Care* 5, no. 1 (2016). longdom.org/open-access/stretching-or-core-strengthening-exercises-for-managing-primary-dysmenorrhea-2167-0420-1000295.pdf.

Walsh, Sally, Elgerta Ismaili, Bushra Naheed, and Shaugn O'Brien. "Diagnosis, Pathophysiology and Management of Premenstrual Syndrome." *The Obstetrician & Gynaecologist* 17, no. 2 (2015): 99–104. doi.org/10.1111/tog.12180.

Wang, L., X. Wang, W. Wang, C. Chen, A. G. Ronnennberg, W. Guang, A. Huang et al. "Stress and Dysmenorrhea: A Population Based Prospective Study." *Occupational Environmental Medicine* 61, no. 12 (2004): 1021–26. doi.org/1136/oem.2003.012302.

Wang, Yi-Xin, Mariel Arvizu, Janet W. Rich-Edwards, Jennifer J. Stuart, JoAnn E. Manson, Stacey A. Missmer, An Pan et al. "Menstrual Cycle Regularity and Length Across the Reproductive Lifespan and Risk of Premature Mortality: Prospective Cohort Study." *BMJ* 371 (2020): m3464. doi.org/10.1136/bmj.m3464.

Zouboulis, Christos C. "The Skin as an Endocrine Organ." *Dermato-endocrinology* 1, no. 5. (2009): 250–52. doi.org/10.4161/derm.1.5.9499.

CHAPTER 7
PREOVULATORY PHASE

Arslan, Ruben C., Katharina M. Schilling, Tanja M. Gerlach, and Lars Penke. "Using 26,000 Diary Entries to Show Ovulatory Changes in Sexual Desire and Behavior." *Journal of Personality and Social Psychology* 121, no. 2 (2018): 410–31. doi.org/10.1037/pspp0000208.

Baerwald, Angela R., Gregg P. Adams, and Roger A. Pierson. "Ovarian Antral Folliculogenesis During the Human Menstrual Cycle: A Review." *Human Reproduction Update* 18, no. 1 (2012): 73–91. doi.org/10.1093/humupd/dmr039.

Bobel, Chris. *New Blood: Third-Wave Feminism and the Politics of Menstruation*. New Jersey: Rutgers University Press, 2010.

Davidsen, L., B. Vistisen, and A. Astrup. "Impact of the Menstrual Cycle on Determinants of Energy Balance: A Putative Role in Weight Loss Attempts." *International Journal of Obesity* 31, no. 12 (2007): 1777–85. doi.org/10.1038/sj.ijo.0803699.

Dunlop, Cheryl E., and Richard A. Anderson. "The Regulation and Assessment of Follicular Growth." *Scandinavian Journal of Clinical and Laboratory Investigation. Supplementum* 244 (2014): 13–17. doi.org/10.3109/00365513.2014.936674.

Erickson, Gregory F. "Follicle Growth and Development." *The Global Library of Women's Medicine* (2008). glowm.com/section-view/heading/follicle-growth-and-development/item/288#.YYr_oGDMIuU.

Figueiro, Mariana G., Bryan Steverson, Judith Heerwagen, Kevin Kampschroer, Claudia M. Hunter, Kassandra Gonzales, Barbara Plitnick et al. "The Impact of Daytime Light Exposures on Sleep and Mood in Office Workers." *Sleep Health* 3, no. 3 (2017): 204–15. doi.org/10.1016/j.sleh.2017.03.005.

Garza, Keli, Kimberly Ann Johnson, Raquel Lemus, and Zhaleh Boyd Phillips. "Fourth Trimester Vaginal Steaming: A Foundational Study." In *Fourth Trimester Vaginal Steaming: A Foundational Study* (2020). fourthtrimestervaginalsteamstudy.com.

Geiker, Nina R.W., Christian Ritz, Sue D. Pedersen, Thomas M. Larsen, James O. Hill, and Arne Astrup. "A Weight-Loss Program Adapted to the Menstrual Cycle Increases Weight Loss in Healthy, Overweight, Premenopausal Women: A 6-mo Randomized Controlled Trial." *American Journal of Clinical Nutrition* 104, no. 1 (2016): 15–20. doi.org/10.3945/ajcn.115.126565.

Guilló-Arakistain, Miren. "Challenging Menstrual Normativity: Nonessentialist Body Politics and Feminist Epistemologies of Health." In The Palgrave Handbook of Critical Menstruation Studies, edited by Chris Bobel, Inga T. Winkler, Breanne Fahs, Katie Ann Hasson, Elizabeth Arveda Kissling, and Tomi-Ann Roberts, 869 -83. Singapore: Palgrave Macmillan, 2020.

Gunter, Jen. "Gwyneth Paltrow Says Steam Your Vagina, An OB/GYN Says Don't." *Dr. Jen Gunter* (blog), November 22, 2020. drjengunter.com/2015/01/27/gwyneth-paltrow-says-steam-your-vagina-an-obgyn-says-dont.

Kundu, Parag, Eran Blacher, Eran Elinav, and Sven Pettersson. "Our Gut Microbiome: The Evolving Inner Self." *Cell* 171, no. 7 (2017): 1481–93. doi.org/10.1016/j.cell.2017.11.024.

Lu, Jiayin, Zixu Wang, Jing Cao, Yaoxing Chen, and Yulan Dong. "A Novel and Compact Review on the Role of Oxidative Stress in Female Reproduction." *Reproductive Biology and Endocrinology* 16, no. 1 (2018): 80. doi.org/10.1186/s12958-018-0391-5.

Mason, Ashley E., Elissa S. Epel, Jean Kristeller, Patricia J. Moran, Mary Dallman, Robert H. Lustig, Michael Acree et al. "Effects of a Mindfulness-Based Intervention on Mindful Eating, Sweets Consumption, and Fasting Glucose Levels in Obese Adults: Data from the SHINE Randomized Controlled Trial." *Journal of Behavioral Medicine* 39, no. 2 (2016): 201–13. doi.org/10.1007/s10865-015-9692-8.

Mikhael, Sasha, Advaita Punjala-Patel, and Larisa Gavrilova-Jordan. "Hypothalamic-Pituitary-Ovarian Axis Disorders Impacting Female Fertility." *Biomedicines* 7, no. 1 (2019): 5. doi.org/10.3390/biomedicines7010005.

Nowak, Debra A., Denise C. Snyder, Ann J. Brown, and Wendy Demark-Wahnefried. "The Effect of Flaxseed Supplementation on Hormonal Levels Associated with Polycystic Ovarian Syndrome: A Case Study." *Current Topics In Nutraceutical Research* 5, no. 4 (2007): 177–81. ncbi.nlm.nih.gov/pmc/articles/PMC2752973.

Sen, Aritro, Hen Prizant, Allison Light, Anindita Biswas, Emily Hayes, Ho-Joon Lee, David Barad et al. "Androgens Regulate Ovarian Follicular Development by Increasing Follicle Stimulating Hormone Receptor and microRNA-125b Expression." *Proceedings of the National Academy of Sciences* 111, no. 8 (2014): 3008–13. doi.org/10.1073/pnas.1318978111.

Toler, Sarah. "Seed Cycling: I Tried It. (And Dug Into the Research on Whether It Works.)" Hello Clue, November 22, 2020. helloclue.com/articles/culture/seed-cycling-i-tried-it-and-dug-into-the-research-on-whether-it-works.

Vandenburg, Tycho, and Virginia Braun. "'Basically, It's Sorcery for your Vagina': Unpacking Western Representations of Vaginal Steaming." *Culture, Health & Sexuality* 19, no. 4 (2017): 470–85. doi.org/10.1080/13691058.2016.1237674.

Wikström-Frisén, Lisbeth, Carl J. Boraxbekk, and Karin Henriksson-Larsén. "Effects on Power, Strength and Lean Body Mass of Menstrual/Oral Contraceptives Cycle Based Resistance Training." *Journal Sports Medicine and Physical Fitness* 57, no. 1–2 (2017): 43–52. doi.org/10.23736/S0022-4707.16.05848-5.

CHAPTER 8
OVULATORY PHASE

Banai, Irena Pavela. "Voice in Different Phases of Menstrual Cycle Among Naturally Cycling Women and Users of Hormonal Contraceptives." *PLOS One* 12, no. 18 (2017): e0183462. doi.org/10.1371/journal.pone.0183462.

Bouchard, Thomas, Len Blackwell, Simon Brown, Richard Fehring, and Suzanne Parenteau-Carreau. "Dissociation Between Cervical Mucus and Urinary Hormones during the Postpartum Return of Fertility in Breastfeeding Women." *The Linacre Quarterly* 85, no. 4 (2018): 399–411. doi.org/10.1177/0024363918809698.

Chevalier, Gaétan, Stephen T. Sinatra, James L. Oschman, Karol Sokal, and Pawel Sokal. "Earthing: Health Implications of Reconnecting the Human Body to the Earth's Surface Electrons." *Journal of Environmental and Public Health* 2012 (2012). doi.org/10.1155/2012/291541.

Chidi-Ogbolu, Nkechinyere, and Keith Baar. "Effect of Estrogen on Musculoskeletal Performance and Injury Risk." *Frontiers in Physiology* 9, no. 1834 (2019). doi.org/10.3389/phys.2018.0183.4.

Comas-Basté, Oriol, Sònia Sánches-Pérez, Maria Teresa Veciana-Nogués, Mariluz Latorre-Moratalla, and María del Carmen Vidal-Carou. "Histamine Intolerance: The Current State of the Art." *Biomolecules* 10, no. 8 (2020): 1181. doi.org/10.3390/biom10081181.

Druet, Anna. "Ovulation Pain 101." Hello Clue, 2019, May 22. helloclue.com/articles/cycle-a-z/ovulation-pain-101.

Fredrickson, Barbara. "Are You Getting Enough Positivity in your Diet?" *Greater Good Magazine*, June 21, 2011. greatergood.berkeley.edu/article/item/are_you_getting_enough_positivity_in_your_diet.

Gentle, Brooke N., Elizabeth G. Pillsworth, and Aaron T. Goetz. "Changes in Sleep Time and Sleep Quality Across the Ovulatory Cycle as a Function of Fertility and Partner Attractiveness." *PLOS One* 9, no. 4 (2014): e92796. doi.org/10.1371/journal.pone.0092796.

Gudmundsdottir, Sigridur Lara, W. Dana Flanders, and Liv Berit Augestad. "Menstrual Cycle Abnormalities in Healthy Women with Low Physical Activity. The North-Trøndelag Population-Based Health Study." *Journal of Physical Activity & Health* 11, no. 6 (2014): 1133–140. doi.org/10.1123/jpah.2012-0284.

Hakimi, Osnat, and Luiz-Claudio Cameron. "Effect of Exercise on Ovulation: A Systematic Review." *Sports Medicine* 47, no. 8 (2017): 1555–567. doi.org/10.1007/s40279-016-0669-8.

Herzberg, Simone D., Makalapua L. Motu'apuaka, William Lambert, Rongwei Fu, Jacqueline Brady, and Jeanne-Marie Guise. "The Effect of Menstrual Cycle and Contraceptives on ACL Injuries and Laxity: A Systematic Review and Meta-Analysis." *Orthopaedic Journal of Sports Medicine* 5, no. 7 (2017). doi.org/10.1177/2325967117718781.

Holder, Mary K, and Jessica A. Mong. "The Role of Ovarian Hormones and the Medial Amygdala in Sexual Motivation." *Current Sexual Health Reports* 9, no. 4 (2017): 262–70. doi.org/10.1007/s11930-017-0131-4.

Mena, Gabriela P., Gregore I. Mielke, and Wendy J. Brown. "The Effect of Physical Activity on Reproductive Health Outcomes in Young Women: A Systematic Review and Meta-Analysis." *Human Reproduction Update* 25, no. 5 (2019): 542–64. doi.org/10.1093/humupd/dmz013.

Menigoz, Wendy, Tracy T. Latz, Robin A. Ely, Cimone Kamei, Gregory Melvin, and Drew Sinatra. "Integrative and Lifestyle Medicine Strategies Should Include Earthing (Grounding): Review of Research Evidence and Clinical Observations." *Explore* 16, no. 3 (2020): 152–60. doi.org/10.1016/j.explore.2019.10.005.

Olesky, Łukasz, Dorota Bylina, Anna Mika, Jaroslaw Soltan, and Renata Kielnar. "The Relationship Between Lumbo-Pelvic-Hip Complex and Knee Joint Dysfunctions." *Journal of Novel Physiotherapies* 8, no. 1 (2018): e149. doi.org/10.4172/2165-7025.1000e149.

Prior, Jerilynn Celia. "How Can We Protect Peak Bone Mass and Future Bone Health for Adolescent Women? By Supporting Ovulation and Avoiding Combined Hormonal Contraceptive Use." *Revista Paulista de Pediatria* 35, no. 2 (2017): 121–24. doi.org/10.1590/1984-0462/;2017;35;2;00019.

Rebollar, Ana Ocampo, Francisco J. Menéndez Balaña, and Montserrat Conde Pastor. "Comparison of Affect Changes during the Ovulatory Phase in Women with and without Hormonal Contraceptives." *Heliyon* 3, no. 4 (2017). doi.org/10.1016/j.heliyon.2017.e00282.

Stein, K. R. van, B. Strauß, and K. Brenk-Franz. "Ovulatory Shifts in Sexual Desire But Not Mate Preferences: An LH-Test-Confirmed, Longitudinal Study." *Evolutionary Psychology* 17, no. 2 (2019). doi.org/10.1177/1474704919848116.

Su, Hsiu-Wei, Yu-Chiao Yi, Ting-Yen Wei, Ting-Chang Chang, and Chao-Min Cheng.

"Detection of Ovulation, A Review of Currently Available Methods." *Bioengineering & Translational Medicine* 2, no. 3 (2017): 238–46. doi.org/10.1002/btm2.10058.

Vigil, Pilar, Carolina Lyon, Betsi Flores, Hernán Rioseco, and Felipe Serrano. "Ovulation, A Sign of Health." *The Linacre Quarterly* 84, no. 4 (2017): 343–55. doi.org/10.1080/00243 639.2017.1394053.

Wilcox, Allen J., David Dunson, and Donna Day Baird. "The Timing of the 'Fertile Window' in the Menstrual Cycle: Day Specific Estimates from a Prospective Study." *BMJ* 321, no. 7271 (2000): 1259–62. doi.org/10.1136/bmj.321.7271.1259.

CHAPTER 9
LUTEAL PHASE

Baker, Fiona C., and Helen S. Driver. "Circadian Rhythms, Sleep, and the Menstrual Cycle." *Sleep Medicine* 8, no 6 (2007): 613–22. doi.org/10.1016/j.sleep.2006.09.011.

Baker, James M., Layla Al-Nakkash, and Melissa M. Herbst-Kralovetz. "Estrogen–Gut Microbiome Axis: Physiological and Clinical Implications." *Maturitas* 103 (2017): 45–53. doi.org/10.1016/j.maturitas.2017.06.025.

Barrett, Lisa Feldman. "PMS Is Not Just a Cliché." *New York Times*, June 8, 2019. nytimes.com/2019/06/08/opinion/sunday/pms.html.

Barth, Claudia, Arno Villringer, and Julia Sacher. "Sex Hormones Affect Neurotransmitters and Shape the Adult Female Brain During Hormonal Transition Periods." *Frontiers in Neuroscience* 9, no. 37 (2015). doi.org/10.3389/fnins.2015.00037.

Bellingrath, Silja, and Brigitte M. Kudielka. "Effort-Reward-Imbalance and Overcommitment are Associated with Hypothalamus-Pituitary-Adrenal (HPA) Axis Responses to Acute Psychosocial Stress in Healthy Working Schoolteachers." *Psychoneuroendocrinology* 33, no. 10 (2008): 1335–43. doi.org/10.1016/j.psyneuen.2008.07.008.

Bloom, Ester. "How 'Treat Yourself' Became a Capitalist Command." *The Atlantic*, November 19, 2015. theatlantic.com/business/archive/2015/11/how-treat-yourself-became-a-consumerist-command/416664.

Chung, Monica S., Laurice Bou Nemer, and Bruce R. Carr. "Does Luteal Phase Deficiency Exist and What Is Its Association with Infertility?" *Reproductive Medicine International* 1, no. 1 (2018). doi.org/10.23937/rmi-2017/1710002.

Cytowic, Richard E. "Stressed Out? Science Says Look at Some Trees." *Psychology Today*, May 16, 2016. psychologytoday.com/us/blog/the-fallible-mind/201605/stressed-out-science-says-look-some-trees.

Deligdisch, Liane. "Hormonal Pathology of the Endometrium." *Modern Pathology* 13, no. 3 (2000): 285–94. doi.org/10.1038/modpathol.3880050.

Draper, C. F., K. Duisters, B. Weger, A. Chakrabarti, A. C. Harms, L. Brennan, T. Hankemeier et al. "Menstrual Cycle Rhythmicity: Metabolic Patterns in Healthy Women." *Scientific Reports* 8, no. 14568 (2018). doi.org/10.1038/s41598-018-32647-0.

Engman, Jonas, Inger Sundström Poromaa, Lena Moby, Johan Wikström, Mats Fredrikson, and Malin Gingnell. "Hormonal Cycle and Contraceptive Effects on Amygdala and Salience Resting-State Networks in Women with Previous Affective Side Effects on the Pill." *Neuropsychopharmacology* 43, no. 3 (2018): 555–63. doi.org/10.1038/npp.2017.157.

Fathizadeh, Nahid, Elham Ebrahimi, Mahboubeh Valiani, Naser Tavakoli, and Manizhe Hojat Yar. "Evaluating the Effect of Magnesium and Magnesium Plus Vitamin B6 Supplement on the Severity of Premenstrual Syndrome." *Iranian Journal of Nursing and Midwifery Research* 15, no. 1 (2010): 401–5. ncbi.nlm.nih.gov/pmc/articles/PMC3208934.

Franklin, Teresa R., Kanchana Jagannathan, Reagan R. Wetherill, Barbara Johnson, Shannon Kelly, Jamison Langguth, Joel Mumma, and Anna Rose Childress. "Influence of Menstrual Cycle Phase on Neural and Craving Responses to Appetitive Smoking Cues in Naturally Cycling Females." *Nicotine & Tobacco Research* 17, no. 4 (2015): 390–97. doi.org/10.1093/ntr/ntu183.

Gibson, Mark. "Corpus Luteum." In *The Global Library of Women's Medicine*. UK:GLOW, 2008. doi.org/10.3843/GLOWM.10291.

Gladding, Rebecca. "This is Your Brain on Meditation." *Psychology Today*, May 22, 2013. psychologytoday.com/us/blog/use-your-mind-change-your-brain/201305/is-your-brain-meditation.

González-Orozco, Juan Carlos, and Ignacio Camacho-Arroyo. "Progesterone Actions During Central Nervous System Development." *Frontiers in Neuroscience* 13, no. 503 (2019). doi.org/10.3389/fnins.2019.00503.

Gröber, Uwe. "Magnesium and Drugs." *International Journal of Molecular Sciences* 20, no. 9 (2019): 2094. doi.org/10.3390/ijms20092094.

Hamilton, Kristen P., Rena Zelig, Anna R. Parker, and Amina Haggag. "Insulin Resistance and Serum Magnesium Concentrations among Women with Polycystic Ovary Syndrome" *Current Developments in Nutrition* 3, no. 11 (2019). doi.org/10.1093/cdn/nzz108.

Hantsoo, Liisa, and C. Neill Epperson. "Premenstrual Dysphoric Disorder: Epidemiology and Treatment." *Current Psychiatry Reports* 17, no. 11 (2015): 87. doi.org/10.1007/s11920-015-0628-3.

Hoerster, Katherine D., Joan C. Chrisler, and Jennifer Gorman Rose. "Attitudes Toward and Experience with Menstruation in the US and India." *Women & Health* 38, no. 3 (2003): 77–95. doi.org/10.1300/J013v38n03_06.

Hormes, Julia M., and Martha A. Niemiec. "Does Culture Create Craving? Evidence from the Case of Menstrual Chocolate Craving." *PLOS One* 12, no. 7 (2017). doi.org/10.1371/journal.pone.0181445.

Hormes, Julia M., and Paul Rozin. "Perimenstrual Chocolate Craving: What Happens After Menopause?" *Appetite* 53, no. 2 (2009): 256–59. doi.org/10.1016/j.appet.2009.07.003.

Joo, Jaehyun, Sinead A. Williamson, Ana I. Vazquez, Jose R. Fernandez, and Molly S. Bray. "The Influence of 15-Week Exercise Training on Dietary Patterns Among Young Adults." *International Journal of Obesity* 43 (2019): 1681–90. doi.org/10.1038/s41366-018-0299-3.

Kwa, Maryann, Claudia S. Plottel, Martin J. Blaser, and Sylvia Adams. "The Intestinal Microbiome and Estrogen Receptor–Positive Female Breast Cancer." *Journal of The National Cancer Institute* 108, no. 8 (2016). doi.org/10.1093/jnci/djw029.

Kwon, Chan-Young, Ik-Hyun Cho, and Kyoung Sun Park. "Therapeutic Effects and Mechanisms of Herbal Medicines for Treating Polycystic Ovary Syndrome: A Review." *Frontiers in Pharmacology* 11 (2020): 1192. doi.org/10.3389/fphar.2020.01192.

Lang, Martin, Jan Krátký, John H. Shaver, Danijela Jerotijević, and Dimitris Xygalatas. "Effects of Anxiety on Spontaneous Ritualized Behavior." *Current Biology* 25, no. 14. (2015): 1892–97. doi.org/10.1016/j.cub.2015.05.049.

Matsumoto, Tamaki, Miho Egawa, Tetsuya Kimura, and Tatsuya Hayashi. "A Potential Relation Between Premenstrual Symptoms and Subjective Perception of Health and Stress Among College Students: A Cross-Sectional Study." *BioPsychoSocial Medicine* 13, no. 26 (2019). doi.org/10.1186/s13030-019-0167-y.

Meenakumari, K. J., S. Agarwal, A. Krishna, and L. K. Pandey. "Effects of Metformin Treatment on Luteal Phase Progesterone Concentration in Polycystic Ovary Syndrome." *Brazilian Journal Medical Biological Research* 37, no. 11 (2004): 1637–44. doi.org/10.1590/s0100-879x2004001100007.

Miller, Paul B., and Michael R. Soules. "Luteal Phase Deficiency: Pathophysiology, Diagnosis, and Treatment," In *The Global Library of Women's Medicine*. GLOWM, 2009. glowm.com/section-view/heading/luteal-phase-deficiency-pathophysiology-diagnosis-and-treatment/item/326#.YZLvZdDMIuU.

Mumford, Sunni L., Jorge E. Chavarro, Cuilin Zhang, Neil J. Perkins, Lindsey A. Sjaarda, Anna Z. Pollack, Karen C. Schliep et al. "Dietary Fat Intake and Reproductive Hormone Concentrations and Ovulation in Regularly Menstruating Women." *American Journal of Clinical Nutrition* 103, no. 3 (2016): 868–77. doi.org/10.3945/ajcn.115.119321.

Parazzini, Fabio, Mirella Di Martino, and Paolo Pellegrino. "Magnesium in the Gynecological Practice: A Literature Review." *Magnesium Research* 30, no. 1 (2017): 1–7. doi.org/10.1684/mrh.2017.0419.

Practice Committee of the American Society for Reproductive Medicine. "Current Clinical Irrelevance of Luteal Phase Deficiency: A Committee Opinion." *Fertility and Sterility* 103, no. 4 (2015): 27–32. doi.org/10.1016/j.fertnstert.2014.12.128.

Reed, Beverly G., and Bruce R. Carr. "The Normal Menstrual Cycle and the Control of Ovulation." *Endotext* (2000). ncbi.nlm.nih.gov/books/NBK279054.

Reimann, Mareike. "The Moderating Role of Overcommitment in the Relationship Between Psychological Contract Breach and Employee Mental Health." *Journal of Occupational Health* 58, no. 5 (2016): 425–33. doi.org/10.1539/joh.16-0032-OA.

Romans, Sarah, Rose Clarkson, Gillian Einstein, Michele Petrovic, and Donna Stewart. "Mood and the Menstrual Cycle: A Review of Prospective Data Studies." *Gender Medicine* 9, no. 5 (2012): 361–84. doi.org/10.1016/j.genm.2012.07.003.

Ryan, Bartholomew. "Manifesto for Maintenance: A Conversation with Mierle Laderman Ukeles." *Art in America*, March 18, 2009. artnews.com/art-in-america/interviews/draft-mierle-interview-56056.

Samavat, Hamed, and Mindy S. Kurzer. "Estrogen Metabolism and Breast Cancer." *Cancer Letters* 356 (no. 2 Pt A) (2015): 231–43. doi.org/10.1016/j.canlet.2014.04.018.

Schliep, Karen C., Sunni L. Mumford, Ahmad O. Hammoud, Joseph B. Stanford, Kerri A. Kissell, Lindsey A. Sjaarda, Neil J. Perkins et al. "Luteal Phase Deficiency in Regularly Menstruating Women: Prevalence and Overlap in Identification Based on Clinical and Biochemical Diagnostic Criteria." *Journal of Clinical Endocrinology & Metabolism* 99, no. 6 (2014): 1007–14. doi.org/10.1210/jc.2013-3534.

Seippel, Lena, and Torbjörn Bäckström. "Luteal-Phase Estradiol Relates to Symptom Severity in Patients with Premenstrual Syndrome." *Journal of Clinical Endocrinology & Metabolism* 83, no. 6. (1998): 1988–92. doi.org/10.1210/jcem.83.6.4899.

Soliman, Ghada A. "Dietary Cholesterol and the Lack of Evidence in Cardiovascular Disease." *Nutrients* 10, no. 6 (2018): 780. doi.org/10.3390/nu10060780.

Takasaki, Akihisa, Hiroshi Tamura, Ken Taniguchi, Hiromi Asada, Toshiaki Taketani, Aki Matsuoka, Yoshiaki Yamagata et al. "Luteal Blood Flow and Luteal Function." *Journal of Ovarian Research* 2, no. 1 (2009). doi.org/10.1186/1757-2215-2-1.

Ussher, Jane. "Premenstrual Syndrome and Self-Policing: Ruptures in Self-Silencing Leading to Increased Self-Surveillance and Blaming of the Body." *Social Theory & Health* 2 (2004): 254–72. doi.org/10.1057/palgrave.sth.8700032.

Uwitonze, Anne Marie, and Mohammed S. Razzaque. "Role of Magnesium in Vitamin D Activation and Function." *Journal of the American Osteopathic Association* 118, no. 3 (2018): 181–89. doi.org/10.7556/jaoa.2018.037.

Vaghela, Nirav, Daxa Mishra, Maitri Sheth, and Vyoma Bharat Dani. "To Compare the Effects of Aerobic Exercise and Yoga on Premenstrual Syndrome." *Journal of Education and Health Promotion* 8 (2019): 199. pubmed.ncbi.nlm.nih.gov/31867375/.

Van den Berg, Magdalena M.H.E., Jolanda Maas, Rianne Muller, Anoek Braun, Wendy Kaandorp, René van Lien, Mireille N.M. van Poppel et al. "Autonomic Nervous System Responses to Viewing Green and Built Setting: Differentiating Between Sympathetic and Parasympathetic Activity." *International Journal of Environmental Research and Public Health* 12, no. 12 (2015): 15860–74. doi.org/10.3390/ijerph121215026.

Van Wingen, G.A., F. van Broekhoven, R. J. Verkes, K. M. Petersson, T. Bäckström, J.K. Buitelaar, and G. Fernández. "Progesterone Selectively Increases Amygdala Reactivity in Women." *Molecular Psychiatry* 13, no. 3 (2008): 325–33. doi.org/10.1038/sj.mp.4002030.

Zhuang, Jin-Ying, Jia-Xi Wang, Qin Lei, Weidong Zhang, and Mingxia Fan. "Neural Basis of Increased Cognitive Control of Impulsivity During the Mid-Luteal Phase Relative to the Late Follicular Phase of the Menstrual Cycle." *Frontiers in Human Neuroscience* 14 (2020): 568399. doi.org/10.3389/fnhum.2020.568399.

CHAPTER 10
MENARCHE

American Academy of Orthopedic Surgeons. "Cushioned Heel Running Shoes May Alter Adolescent Biomechanics, Performance." *ScienceDaily*, March 19, 2013. sciencedaily.com/releases/2013/03/130319091420.htm.

Cense, Marianne. "Rethinking Sexual Agency: Proposing a Multicomponent Model Based on Young People's Life Stories." *Sex Education* 19, no. 3 (2019): 247–62. doi.org/10.1080/14681811.2018.1535968.

Chrisler, Joan C., and Ingrid Johnston-Robledo. *Woman's Embodied Self: Feminist Perspectives on Identity and Image*. Washington, DC: American Psychological Association, 2018.

DiCesare, Christopher A., Alicia Montalvo, Kim D. Barber Foss, Staci M. Thomas, Kevin R. Ford, Timothy E. Hewett, Neeru A. Jayanthi et al. "Lower Extremity Biomechanics Are Altered Across Maturation in Sport-Specialized Female Adolescent Athletes." *Frontiers in Pediatric*s 7 (2019): 268. doi.org/10.3389/fped.2019.00268.

Leung, Hildie, Daniel T. L. Shek, Edvina Leung, and Esther Y. W. Shek. "Development of Contextually-Relevant Sexuality Education: Lessons from a Comprehensive Review of Adolescent Sexuality Education Across Cultures." *International Journal of Environmental Research and Public Health* 16, no. 4 (2019): 621. doi.org/10.3390/ijerph16040621.

Lower, Jacinta, and Marika Tiggemann. "Body Dissatisfaction, Dieting Awareness and the Impact of Parental Influence in Young Children." *British Journal of Health Psychology* 8, no. 2 (2010): 135–47. doi.org/10.1348/135910703321649123.

McHugh, Maureen C. "Menstrual Shame: Exploring the Role of 'Menstrual Moaning.'" In *The Palgrave Handbook of Critical Menstruation* Studies, edited by Chris Bobel, Inga T. Winkler, Breanne Fahs, Katie Ann Hasson, Elizabeth Arveda Kissling, and Tomi-Ann Roberts, 409–22. Singapore: Palgrave Macmillan, 2020. doi.org/10.1007/978-981-15-0614-7_32.

Meland, Eivind, Siren Haugland, and Hans-Johan Breidablik. "Body Image and Perceived Health in Adolescence." *Health Education Research* 22, no. 3 (2007): 342–50. doi.org/10.1093/her/cyl085.

Moschonis, George, Dimitrois Papandreou, Christina Mavrogianni, Angeliki Giannopoulou, Louisa Damianidi, Pavlos Malindretos et al. "Association of Iron Depletion with Menstruation and Dietary Intake Indices in Pubertal Girls: The Healthy Growth Study." *BioMed Research International* 2013 (2013). doi.org/10.1155/2013/423263.

Nuefeld, Karen-Anne McVey, Pauline Luczynski, Timothy G. Dinan, and John F. Cryan. "Reframing the Teenage Wasteland: Adolescent Microbiota-Gut-Brain Axis." *Canadian Journal of Psychiatry* 61, no. 4 (2016): 214–21. doi.org/10.1177/0706743716635536.

Provensi, Gustavo, Scheila D. Schmidt, Marcus Boehme, Thomaz F. S. Bastiaanssen, Barbara Rani, Alessia Costa, Kizkirza Busca et al. "Preventing Adolescent Stress-Induced Cognitive and Microbiome Changes by Diet." *PNAS* 116, no. 19 (2019): 9644–51. doi.org/10.1073/pnas.1820832116.

Schooler, Deborah, L. Monique Ward, Ann Merriweather, and Allison S. Caruthers.

"Cycles of Shame: Menstrual Shame, Body Shame, and Sexual Decision-Making."
Journal of Sex Research 42, no. 4 (2005): 324–34. jstor.org/stable/3813785.

Twenge, Jean M., Thomas E. Joiner, Megan L. Rogers, and Gabrielle N. Martin.
"Increases in Depressive Symptoms, Suicide-Related Outcomes, and Suicide Rates
Among U.S. Adolescents After 2010 and Links to Increased New Media Screen Time."
Clinical Psychological Science 6, no. 1 (2017): 3–17. doi.org/10.1177/2167702617723376.

White, Mathew P., Ian Alcock, James Grellier, Benedict W. Wheeler, Terry Hartig, Sara
L. Warber, Angie Bone et al. "Spending at Least 120 Minutes a Week in Nature is
Associated with Good Health and Wellbeing." *Scientific Reports* 9, no. 7730 (2019). doi.
org/10.1038/s41598-019-44097-3.

CHAPTER 11
THE MENSTRUATING YEARS

Barzilai-Pesach, Vered, Einat K. Sheiner, Eyal Sheiner, Gad Potashnik, and Ilana
Shoham-Vardi. "The Effect of Women's Occupational Psychological Stress on Outcome
of Fertility Treatments." *Journal of Occupational Environmental Medicine* 48, no. 1
(2006): 56–62. doi.org/10.1097/01.jom.0000183099.47127.e9.

Brawn, Jennifer, Matteo Morotti, Krina T. Zondervan, Christian M. Becker, and Katy
Vincent. "Central Changes Associated with Chronic Pelvic Pain and Endometriosis."
Human Reproduction Update 20, no. 5 (2014): 737–47. doi.org/10.1093/humupd/
dmu025.

Gaskins, Audrey J., and Jorge E. Chavarro. "Diet and Fertility: A Review." *American
Journal of Obstetrics and Gynecology* 218, no. 4 (2018): 379–89. doi.org/10.1016/j.
ajog.2017.08.010.

Gerritsen, Roderik J. S., and Guido P. H. Band. "Breath of Life: The Respiratory Vagal
Stimulation Model of Contemplative Activity." *Frontiers in Human Neuroscience* 12, no.
397 (2018). doi.org/10.3389/fnhum.2018.00397.

Győrffy, Zsuzsa, Diána Dweik, and Edmond Girasek. "Reproductive Health and Burnout Among Female Physicians: Nationwide, Representative Study from Hungary." *BMC
Women's Health* 14, no. 121 (2014). doi.org/10.1186/1472-6874-14-121.

Hamidovic, Ajna, Kristina Karapetyan, Fadila Serdarevic, So Hee Choi, Tory Eisenlohr-
Moul, and Graziano Pinna. "Higher Circulating Cortisol in the Follicular vs. Luteal Phase
of the Menstrual Cycle: A Meta-Analysis." *Frontiers in Endocrinology* 11, no. 311 (2020).
doi.org/10.3389/fendo.2020.00311.

Hannibal, Kara E., and Mark D. Bishop. "Chronic Stress, Cortisol Dysfunction, and Pain:

A Psychoneuroendocrine Rationale for Stress Management and Pain Rehabilitation." *Physical Therapy* 94, no. 12 (2014): 1816–25. doi.org/10.2522/ptj.20130597.

Koch, Liz. *Stalking Wild Psoas: Embodying Your Core Intelligence.* Berkeley, CA: North Atlantic Books, 2019.

Korsmo, Hunter W., Xinyin Jiang, and Marie A. Caudill. "Choline: Exploring the Growing Science on Its Benefits for Moms and Babies." *Nutrients* 11, no. 8 (2019): 1823. doi.org/10.3390/nu11081823.

Lopez, Barry. "The Invitation." *Granta,* November 18, 2015. granta.com/invitation.

Mills, J. L., G. M. Buck Louis, K. Kannan, J. Weck, Y. Wan, J. Maisog, A. Giannakou et al. "Delayed Conception in Women with Low-Urinary Iodine Concentrations: A Population-Based Prospective Cohort Study." *Human Reproduction* 33, no. 3 (2018): 426–33. doi.org/10.1093/humrep/dex379.

Nagoski, Emily, and Amelia Nagoski. *Burnout: The Secret to Unlocking the Stress Cycle.* New York: Ballantine Books, 2020.

Paananen, Markus, Peter O'Sullivan, Leon Straker, Darren Beales, Pieter Coenen, Jaro Karppinen, Craig Pennel et al. "A Low Cortisol Response to Stress is Associated with Musculoskeletal Pain Combined with Increased Pain Sensitivity in Young Adults: A Longitudinal Cohort Study." *Arthritis Research & Therapy* 17, no. 355 (2015). doi.org/10.1186/s13075-015-0875-z.

Purvanova, Radostina K., and John P. Muros. "Gender Differences in Burnout: A Meta-Analysis." *Journal of Vocational Behavior* 77, no. 2 (2010): 168–85. doi.org/10.1016/j.jvb.2010.04.006.

Rooney, Kristin L., and Alice D. Domar. "The Relationship Between Stress and Infertility." *Dialogues in Clinical Neuroscience* 20, no. 1 (2018): 41–47. doi.org/10.31887/DCNS.2018.20.1/klrooney.

Salvagioni, Denise Albieri Jodas, Francine Nessello Melanda, Arthur Eumann Mesas, Alberto Durán González, Flávia Lopes Gabani, and Selma Maffei de Andrade. "Physical, Psychological and Occupational Consequences of Job Burnout: A Systematic Review of Prospective Studies." *PLOS One* 12, no. 10 (2017). doi.org/10.1371/journal.pone.0185781.

Staugaard-Jones, Jo Ann. *The Vital Psoas Muscle: Connecting Physical, Emotional, and Spiritual Well-Being.* Berkeley, CA: North Atlantic Books, 2012.

Stothard, Ellen R., Andrew W. McHill, Christopher M. Depner, Brian R. Birks, Thomas M. Moehlman, Hannah K. Ritchie, Jacob R. Guzzetti et al. "Circadian Entrainment to the Natural Light-Dark Cycle Across Seasons and the Weekend." *Current Biology* 27, no. 4 (2017): 508–13. doi.org/10.1016/j.cub.2016.12.041.

Umberson, Debra, and Jennifer Karas Montez. "Social Relationships and Health: A Flashpoint for Health Policy." *Journal of Health and Social Behavior* 51, no. Suppl (2010): 54–66. doi.org/10.1177/0022146510383501.

Wallace, Taylor C., Jan Krzysztof Blusztajn, Marie A. Caudill, Kevin C. Klatt, Elana Natker, Steven H. Zeisel, and Kathleen M. Zelman. "Choline: The Underconsumed and Underappreciated Essential Nutrient." *Nutrition Today* 53, no. 6 (2018): 240–53. doi.org/10.1097/NT.0000000000000302.

Webb, Christine E., Maya Rossignac-Milon, and E. Tory Higgins. "Stepping Forward Together: Could Walking Facilitate Interpersonal Conflict Resolution?" *American Psychology* 72, no. 4 (2017): 374–85. doi.org/10.1037/a0040431.

CHAPTER 12
THE MENOPAUSAL TRANSITION

Almeida, Osvaldo P., Kylie Marsh, Karen Murray, Martha Hickey, Moira Sim, Andrew Ford, and Leon Flicker. "Reducing Depression During the Menopausal Transition with Health Coaching: Results from the Healthy Menopausal Transition Randomised Controlled Trial." *Maturitas* 92 (2016): 41–48. doi.org/10.1016/j.maturitas.2016.07.012.

Barrett, Lisa Feldman. *How Emotions Are Made: The Secret Life of the Brain*. New York: First Mariner Books, 2018.

Barrett, Lisa Feldman. "How Emotions Trick Your Brain." *Science Focus*, May 2018, sciencefocus.com/the-human-body/how-emotions-trick-your-brain-2.

Barrett, Lisa Feldman. "People's Words and Actions Can Actually Shape Your Brain—A Neuroscientist Explains How." *TED Science*, November 17, 2020. ideas.ted.com/peoples-words-and-actions-can-actually-shape-your-brain-a-neuroscientist-explains-how.

Barrett, Lisa Feldman. "The Science of Making Emotions." *Health Watch*, May/June 2018, 38–39.

Barrett, Lisa Feldman. "Your Brain is Not for Thinking." *New York Times*, November 23, 2020. nytimes.com/2020/11/23/opinion/brain-neuroscience-stress.html.

Brinton, Roberta, Jia Yao, Fei Yin, and Wendy Mack. "Perimenopause as a Neurological Transition State." *Nature Reviews Endocrinology* 11 (2015): 393–405. doi.org/10.1038/nrendo.2015.82.

Chapman, Simon N., Jenni E. Pettay, Virpi Lummaa, and Mirkka Lahdenperä. "Limits to Fitness Benefits of Prolonged Post-Reproductive Life in Women." *Current Biology* 29, no. 4 (2019): 645–50. doi.org/10.1016/j.cub.2018.12.052.

Daubenmier, Jennifer, Patricia J. Moran, Jean Kristeller, Michael Acree, Peter Bacchetti, Margaret E. Kemeny, Mary Dallman et al. "Effects of a Mindfulness-Based Weight Loss Intervention in Adults with Obesity: A Randomized Clinical Trial." *Obesity* 24, no. 4 (2016): 794–804. doi.org/10.1002/oby.21396.

de Cabo, Rafael, and Mark P. Mattson. "Effects of Intermittent Fasting on Health, Aging, and Disease." *New England Journal of Medicine* 381 (2019): 2541–51. doi.org/10.1056/NEJMra1905136.

Hall, Lisa, Lynn Clark Callister, Judith A. Berry, and Geraldine Matsumura. "Meanings of Menopause: Cultural Influences on Perception and Management of Menopause." *Journal of Holistic Nursing* 25, no. 2 (2007): 106–18. https://doi.org/10.1177/0898010107299432.

Illing, Sean, and Jamil Smith. "We Don't Just Feel Emotions. We Make Them." Interview with Lisa Feldman Barrett. *Vox Conversations*, Podcast audio, January 6, 2021. open.spotify.com/episode/4GZJ6jzyEqxTdSkWDZOzyl.

Ip, Chi Kin, Lei Zhang, Aitak Farzi, Yue Qi, Ireni Clarke, Felicia Reed, Yan-Chuan Shi et al. "Amygdala NPY Circuits Promote the Development of Accelerated Obesity Under Chronic Stress Conditions." *Cell Metabolism* 30, no. 1 (2019): 111–28. doi.org/10.1016/j.cmet.2019.04.001.

Kimmerer, Robin Wall. "The Serviceberry: An Economy of Abundance." *Emergence Magazine*, December 10, 2020. emergencemagazine.org/story/the-serviceberry.

Kohn, Grace E., Katherine M. Rodriguez, James Hotaling, and Alexander W. Pastuszak. "The History of Estrogen Therapy." *Sexual Medicine Reviews* 7, no. 3 (2019): 416–21. doi.org/10.1016/j.sxmr.2019.03.006.

Kumler, Emily. "Menopause and How Older Women are Essential to Societies." Interview with Kristen Hawkes. *Empowered Health*. Podcast audio. September 9, 2019. empoweredhealthshow.com/kristen-hawkes-grandmother-hypothesis.

Lazar, Amanda, Norman Makoto Su, Jeffrey Bardzell, and Shaowen Bardzell. "Parting the Red Sea: Sociotechnical Systems and Lived Experience of Menopause." *Proceedings of the 2019 CHI Conference on Human Factors in Computing Systems* (2019): 1–16. doi.org/10.1145/3290605.3300710.

Mattern, Susan P. *The Slow Moon Climbs: The Science, History, and Meaning of Menopause*. Princeton, NJ: Princeton University Press, 2019.

Mosconi, Lisa. *The XX Brain: The Groundbreaking Science Empowering Women to Maximize Cognitive Health and Prevent Alzheimer's Disease*. New York, NY: Avery, 2020.

Nattrass, Stuart, Darren P. Croft, Samuel Ellis, Michael A. Cant, Michael N. Weiss, Brianna M. Wright, Eva Stredulinsky et al. "Postreproductive Killer Whale Grandmothers Improve the Survival of Their Grandoffspring." *PNAS* 116, no. 52 (2019): 26669–73. doi.org/10.1073/pnas.1903844116.

Santoro, Nanette. "Perimenopause: From Research to Practice." *Journal of Women's Health* 25, no. 4 (2016): 332–39. doi.org/10.1089/jwh.2015.5556.

Sohn, Emily. "How the Evidence Stacks up for Preventing Alzheimer's Disease." *Nature* 559, no. 7715 (2018): S18–S20. doi.org/10.1038/d41586-018-05724-7.

Speroff, Leon. "The Perimenopause Definitions, Demography, and Physiology." *Obstetrics & Gynecology Clinics of North America* 29, no. 3 (2002): 397–410. doi.org/10.1016/S0889-8545(02)00007-4.

University of Jyväskylä. "Menopause and Estrogen Affect Muscle Function." *ScienceDaily*, October 2, 2017. sciencedaily.com/releases/2017/10/171002085656.htm.

Zhao Di, Chunqin Liu, Xiujuan Feng, Fangyan Hou, Xiaofang Xu, and Ping Li. "Menopausal Symptoms in Different Substages of Perimenopause and Their Relationships with Social Support and Resilience." *Menopause* 26, no. 3 (2019): 233–39. doi.org/10.1097/GME.0000000000001208.

CHAPTER 13
THE POSTMENOPAUSAL YEARS

Alves, Bruna Cherubini, Thaís Rasia da Silva, and Poli Mara Spritzer. "Sedentary Lifestyle and High-Carbohydrate Intake Are Associated with Low-Grade Chronic Inflammation in Post-Menopause: A Cross-Sectional Study." *Revista Brasileira de Ginecoloigia e Obstetretcia*. 38, no. 7 (2016): 317–24. doi.org/10.1055/s-0036-1584582.

Barrett, Lisa Feldman. "How 'Superagers' Stay Sharp in Their Later Years." *The Observer*, April 30, 2017. theguardian.com/science/2017/apr/30/work-on-your-ageing-brain-superagers-mental-excercise-lisa-feldman-barrett.

Buettner, Dan, and Sam Skemp. "Blue Zones: Lessons from the World's Longest Lived." *American Journal of Lifestyle Medicine* 10, no. 5 (2016): 318–21. doi.org/10.1177/1559827616637066.

Cagnacci, Angelo, and Martina Venier. "The Controversial History of Hormone Replacement Therapy." *Medicina* 55, no. 9 (2019): 602. doi.org/10.3390/medicina55090602.

Duckworth, Angela. *Grit: The Power of Passion and Perseverance.* New York: Scribner, 2016.

Duckworth, Angela. "Sleep Success: Setting Yourself Up for New Year's Resolutions." *Character Lab*, January 5, 2020. characterlab.org/tips-of-the-week/sleep-success.

Gangwisch, James E., Lauren Hale, Marie-Pierre St-Onge, Lydia Choi, Erin S. LeBlanc, Dolores Malaspina, Mark G Opler et al. "High Glycemic Index and Glycemic Load Diets as Risk Factors for Insomnia: Analyses from the Women's Health Initiative." *American Journal of Nutrition* 111, no. 2 (2019): 429–39. doi.org/10.1093/ajcn/nqz275.

Gunter, Jennifer. *The Vagina Bible.* New York: Citadel Press Books, 2019.

Kline, Christopher E., Martica H. Hall, Daniel J. Buysse, Conrad P. Earnest, Timothy S. Church. "Poor Sleep Quality Is Associated with Insulin Resistance in Postmenopausal Women With and Without Metabolic Syndrome." *Metabolic Syndrome and Related Disorders* 16, no. 4 (2018): 183–89. doi.org/10.1089/met.2018.0013.

Kroese, Floor M., Catharine Evers, Marieke A. Adriaanse, and Denise T. D. de Ridder. "Bedtime Procrastination: A Self-Regulation Perspective on Sleep Insufficiency in the General Population." *Journal of Health Psychology* 21, no. 5 (2016): 853–62. doi.org/10.1177/1359105314540014.

Masala, G., B. Bendinelli, C. Della Bella, M. Assedi, S. Tapinassi, I. Ermini, D. Occhini et al. "Inflammatory Marker Changes in a 24-month Dietary and Physical Activity Randomised Intervention in Postmenopausal Women." *Scientific Reports* 10, no. 21845 (2020). doi.org/10.1038/s41598-020-78796-z.

Meslier, Victoria, Manolo Laiola, Henrik M. Roager, Francesca De Filippis, Hugo Roume, Benoit Quinquis, Rosalba Giacco et al. "Mediterranean Diet Intervention in Overweight and Obese Subjects Lowers Plasma Cholesterol and Causes Changes in the Gut Microbiome and Metabolome Independently of Energy Intake." *Gut Microbiota* 69, no. 7 (2020): 1258–68. doi.org/10.1136/gutjnl-2019-320438.

Namazi, Masoumeh, Rasoul Sadeghi, and Zahra Behboodi Moghadam. "Social Determinants of Health in Menopause: An Integrative Review." *International Journal of Women's Health* 11 (2019): 637–47. doi.org/10.2147/IJWH.S228594.

Nilsson, Christina, Ingela Lundgren, Annika Karlström, and Ingegerd Hildingsson. "Self Reported Fear of Childbirth and Its Association with Women's Birth Experience and Mode of Delivery: A Longitudinal Population-Based Study." *Women and Birth* 25, no. 3 (2013): 114–21. doi.org/10.1016/j.wombi.2011.06.001.

The North American Menopause Society. "Cognitive Behavioral Therapy Shown to Improve Multiple Menopause Symptoms." *ScienceDaily*, May 29, 2019. sciencedaily.com/releases/2019/05/190529113047.htm.

Paul, Annie Murphy. *The Extended Mind: The Power of Thinking Outside the Brain*. New York: Houghton Mifflin Harcourt, 2021.

Pinkerton, JoAnn V. "Hormone Therapy for Postmenopausal Women." *New England Journal of Medicine* 382, no. 5 (2020): 446–55. doi.org/10.1056/NEJMcp1714787.

Steward, Donna E. "Menopause in Highland Guatemala Mayan Women." *Maturitas* 44, no. 4 (2003): 293–97. doi.org/10.1016/S0378-5122(03)00036-7.

Stoll, Kathrin, and Wendy Hall. "Vicarious Birth Experiences and Childbirth Fear: Does it Matter How Young Canadian Women Learn About Birth?" *Journal of Perinatal Education* 22, no. 4 (2013): 226–33. doi.org/10.1891/1058-1243.22.4.226.

Sun, Felicia W., Michael R. Stepanovic, Joseph Andreano, Lisa Feldman Barrett, Alexandra Touroutoglou, and Bradford C. Dickerson. "Youthful Brains in Older Adults: Preserved Neuroanatomy in the Default Mode and Salience Networks Contributes to Youthful Memory in Superaging." *Journal of Neuroscience* 36, no. 37 (2016): 9659–68. jneurosci.org/content/36/37/9659.

Talbot, Margaret. "Is It Really Too Late to Learn New Skills?" *The New Yorker*, January 11, 2021. newyorker.com/magazine/2021/01/18/is-it-really-too-late-to-learn-new-skills.

Walker, Matthew. *Why We Sleep: Unlocking the Power of Sleep and Dreams*. New York: Scribner, 2017.

Walsh, Dana M., Alexis N. Hokenstad, Jun Chen, Jaeyun Sung, Gregory D. Jenkins, Nicholas Chia, Heidi Nelson et al. "Postmenopause as a Key Factor in the Composition of the Endometrial Cancer Microbiome (ECbiome)." *Scientific Reports* 9, no. 19213 (2019). doi.org/10.1038/s41598-019-55720-8.

Wu, Rachel, George W. Rebok, and Feng Vankee Lin. "A Novel Theoretical Life Course Framework for Triggering Cognitive Development Across the Lifespan." *Human Development* 59, no. 6 (2016): 342–65. www.jstor.org/stable/26765153.

Index

H

Hawkes, Kristen, 233
Hippocrates, 42
"History of Self-Care" (Harris), 40
hormonal contraception, 9–10, 47–49, 132
    birth control pills, 43
    for pain relief, 70, 131
    PMS and, 157
    sexual desire and, 124
    skin conditions and, 75
hormone deficiency disease, 233–34, 235
hormone replacement therapy (HRT), 234–35
hormones, x, 6, 13, 24, 74–75, 100, 159
    cognition and, 27
    disorders of, 17, 131–32
    and hormonal contraception,
        comparison of, 48
    "imbalance" in, 16–17
    movement and health of, 38–39
    in preovulatory phase, 99
    in puberty, 191
    throughout lifecycle (chart), 218–19
How Emotions Are Made (Barret), 223, 225
How to Do Nothing (Odell), 73
human chorionic gonadotropin (hCG), 19, 157
Human Reproduction, 212
hypothalamus-pituitary-adrenal (HPA)axis,
    132, 203
hypothalamic-pituitary-ovarian (HPO) axis,
    13, 67
hypothalamus, role of, 13–14

I

immune system, 29, 74, 93, 99, 118, 167, 198, 203
inflammatory response, 29, 38, 64, 167, 203,
    244, 248
insulin, 33–34
    metabolism, 158
    resistance, 67, 89, 132, 212–13
    sensitivity, 36–37, 99, 101
intelligence, fluid and crystallized, 242
intersexuality, 16
Invisible Women (Perez), 201
iodine, 114, 211, 212
iron, in puberty, 198–99
"Is It Really Too Late to Learn New Skills?"
    (Talbot), 242

J

Jacobi, Mary Putnam, 30, 43
Journal of Environmental and Public Health, 137
Journal of Psychosomatic Obstetrics &
    Gynecology, 204
Journal of Sex Research, 193

K

Kissling, Elizabeth, 64–65, 191
Koch, Liz, 208–9

L

language, 64–65, 166, 188–89
leave, maternity and paternity, 202–3
light exposure, 55, 105, 161, 228
Lopez, Barry, 205
luteal phase, 7, 8, 163
    blood sugar in, 34
    brain during, 162–63
    cervical secretions in, 50, 52
    estrogen in, 158
    movement in, 170–72
    physiology, 66, 154
    PMS and, 154–56
    postpartum, 130
    progesterone in, 19, 159
    at puberty, 191–92
    recipes for, 173–85
    seed cycling in, 100
    self-care in, 163, 167–68
    self-protection in, 28, 29
    transition to, 124, 127
luteinizing hormone (LH), 7, 8, 127–28, 129,
    131, 164, 191

M

male ritualized bleeding, 3–4
Marquette Method, 129
masturbation, 72, 76, 124, 134, 190
Mattern, Susan P., 215, 235, 236, 246
McCallum, Mary, 77, 95, 106, 121, 135, 151,
    169, 185
medical and health professionals, when to
    consult, 132, 156, 157, 158, 226, 248
meditation, 40, 102
Mediterranean diet, 211, 220, 249, 250
menarche, 187, 191

progesterone (*cont.*)
    in HRT, 234–35
    in luteal phase, 7, 157
    in menopausal transition, 217
    nutritional support for, 90
    postpartum, 130
    in thermoregulation and body
        temperature, 54
prolactin, 39, 129
psoas, 208–10
Psychoneuroendocrinology, 163
puberty, 12, 13–14, 18, 98, 191–92. *See also*
    menarche

Q

"Question of Rest for Women During
    Menstruation, The" (Jacobi), 30

R

racism, 21, 25, 40, 44, 202
Ramage, Estelle, 64
recipes, 81
    Ashwagandha Moon Milk, 94
    Berry, Ginger, and Greens Kefir
        Smoothie, 118
    Brothy Pureed White Beans, 175–76
    Chicken and Sweet Potatoes, 84–85
    Chocolate Bark, 183
    Chocolate-Chaga Avocado Pudding, 93
    Collagen-Rich Creamsicle Cups, 92
    Collard Green Spring Rolls, 111–12
    Crispy Pastured Pork Larb, 143–44
    Dandelion Burdock Root Chai, 95
    Follicular Seed Balls, 119
    Grass-Fed Beef Liver, 145
    Hawthorn Rose Syrup, 151
    Kabocha Squash Curry Soup, 173–74
    Lacto-Fermented Carrots, 110
    Lamb Curry, 87–88
    Luteal Seed Balls, 181
    Maple Pear Custard, 184
    Matcha Cacao and Coconut Butter
        Cups, 120
    Mussels with Kale, 114
    Nourishing Blood-Building Tea, 185
    Oatstraw Herbal Latte, 121
    Oven Braised Short Ribs, 176–77

    Oysters, 148
    Plentiful Greens Oat Flour Pancakes, 149
    Purple Sauerkraut, 138
    Quick Pickled Radishes and Carrots, 140
    Roasted Acorn Squash, 178–79
    Roasted Cauliflower, 113
    Roasted Cod and Asparagus, 146–47
    Roasted Pears, 182
    Sardine Cakes, 117
    Smashed Beets and Bitter Greens, 179–
        80
    Snacking Chickpeas, 90–91
    Sprouted Grain-Free Granola, 150
    Stir-Fried Forbidden Rice, 141–42
    Tom Kha Gai, 85–86
    Wakame, Ginger, and Miso Soba
        Noodles, 115–16
    Watercress Salad, 89
    Wild Salmon and Roe Temaki, 139
    Wild Salmon Congee, 82–83
reciprocity, 227–28
reproductive health, xi, 38, 44, 202, 212
resilience, 40–41, 94, 202, 204–5, 221, 226,
    231, 240
rest and sleep, 160–61
    blood sugar and, 35, 37
    earthing for, 137
    light and, 105
    in menopausal transition, 227, 228
    during menstrual phase, 73
    nutritional support for, 94, 248–49
    painful periods and, 72
    in postmenopause, 245, 247
rights, human and reproductive, 1, 5, 11,
    30, 44
Ryan, Timothy, 38

S

Scientific Reports, 197, 244
screen time, 55, 105, 196
seasonal metaphors, ix–x, 59
    fall (luteal phase), 153–54, 163
    life's stages, 187, 221
    spring (preovulatory phase), 97–98,
        99–100
    summer (ovulatory phase), 123–24
    winter (menstrual phase), 60, 63, 64, 73